I WILL DO BETTER

Also by Charles Bock

Beautiful Children
Alice & Oliver

I WILL
DO BETTER

A FATHER'S MEMOIR OF

HEARTBREAK, PARENTING,

AND LOVE

CHARLES BOCK

ABRAMS PRESS, NEW YORK

Library of Congress Control Number: 2024936147

ISBN: 978-1-4197-7442-3
eISBN: 979-8-88707-315-6

Printed and bound in the United States
10 9 8 7 6 5 4 3 2 1

Abrams books are available at special discounts when purchased in quantity for premiums and promotions as well as fundraising or educational use. Special editions can also be created to specification. For details, contact specialsales@abramsbooks.com or the address below.

Abrams Press® is a registered trademark of Harry N. Abrams, Inc.

ABRAMS The Art of Books
195 Broadway, New York, NY 10007
abramsbooks.com

AUTHOR'S NOTE

THIS BOOK WAS written with the aim of conveying the larger and essential truths of what Lily and I experienced together during the first two years after her mother passed. I relied on emails, journals, photos, and documents, researched whatever facts I could, talked with numerous people from this time, and, of course, relied on my own memories. I tried to get things right. The most important names have remained the same. However, I also changed the names and identifying details of some people to protect their privacy. Some characters are composites, combining a number of friends, lovers, etc. Time frames similarly get compressed. Various events have been combined.

To the Reader:

. . . Had my intention been to seek the world's favor, I should surely have adorned myself with borrowed beauties: I desire therein to be viewed as I appear in mine own genuine, simple, and ordinary manner, without study and artifice: for it is myself I paint . . .

—Montaigne, this first day of March, fifteen hundred and eighty.

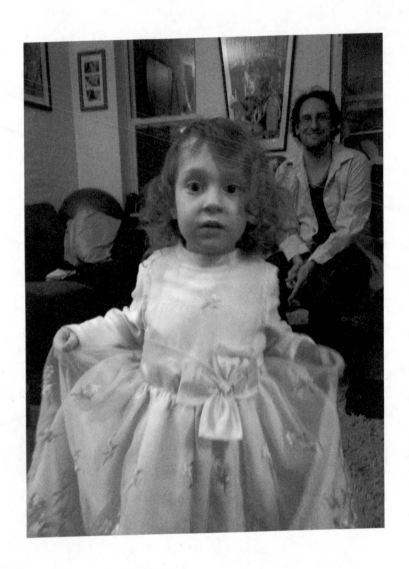

THREE
YEARS OLD

CHAPTER ONE

FROST DUSTED FOURTEENTH Street; the taxi headed eastward, away from the hospital, along the imaginary line that separated downtown from the rest of this dark and morbid city. Three in the morning, December 8. Not a word from the driver. Logistics swam through my head: Lily was staying with her grandmother, Peg, who was in town from Memphis; I'd have to talk with Peg in the morning, make sure Lily's day was occupied—a museum trip, something. I'd have to work on Diana's funeral arrangements. Tired beyond words.

I vaguely remember getting out of the taxi, the pricks of cold like needles on my face. Suitcases and overstuffed trash bags filled the trunk and back seat: Diana's clothes and underwear, her laptop and pill regimen, her prayer journals, her motivational posters, family photos. I struggled to unload everything onto the street, right outside our apartment on Twenty-Second. A neighbor saw me. He was a promoter of gay nightlife, either going to or coming back from a club. Did I need help?

I started to answer, then broke down, going weak in his arms, sobbing onto his shoulder.

Diana had moved into my one-bedroom apartment after we married, but she was adamant: the place was too small for two adults, let alone the addition of a baby. She was anxious to find somewhere better, and though I maintained an unhealthy attachment to my pad—I'd lived there for a decade, it was rent-stabilized, convenient—I agreed to search. We almost moved to a place in Harlem, only they didn't allow dogs, and I couldn't abandon my aged Shih Tzu. Instead, a friend helped me sand the floors, repaint. My dog had to be put down months later. Even with newly painted walls and smooth floors, our apartment remained cramped, tawdry.

Now I stepped back inside. Darkness coated our belongings, everything just like when we'd left: the metal walker still next to Diana's desk, the schedule for the visiting nurse taped to the bedroom door. Silence like a crypt. I accidentally kicked colored wooden blocks scattered along the throw rug.

My God. The weight of this universe.

LILY WAS FOCUSED on one thing, the event Diana had been determined to stay alive for, but had missed by three scant days: *party party party*. Three years old. Daddy's big girl didn't come up to my waist, wasn't close to seeing above the bathroom sink and finding her reflection, couldn't have weighed thirty pounds. This was going to be her first *real* birthday party.

Common sense—belonging to anyone within a blast radius—dictated it would have been cruel to ruin the festivities for her. I concentrated on the tasks at hand: making calls to a woman who ran a funeral home out of her Brooklyn apartment (for a reasonable price she handled the cremation); following up with a Ninth Avenue bakery (confirming the color of the iced letters, the birthday message on the double-chocolate cake). Peg, Diana's mother, was in shock, numb with grief, exhausted by sitting witness to what her only child had been through. The chance to be with Lily—to help her granddaughter—was the only thing keeping her in one piece. She and Diana's friend Susannah helped Lily into a sleeveless formal dress. Lily preened in the midnight blue gown, marveling at the silk flowers around its waist. The frock was a little too big, its hem grazing the floor. Lily twisted in place, swishing the tulle back and forth, giggling at the little rustling sounds. Her face glowed from some inner place, her eyes sizzled gray, their green flecks shining. Ko—the sitter—asked Lily to hold still, dutifully worked Lily's hair into pigtails—wait, there may have been a braid. I seem to remember a braid. Except her hair was so fine that a braid might have been impossible.

My sister, Crystal, supplemented her acting career by planning and working at children's birthday parties. Her West Village apartment easily converted to a wonderland of toys, the perfect celebration spot. When Lily arrived, parents were trying to keep their kids from looting the table of cookies and treats; toddlers were already berserk from sugar, running around, flapping their arms, wrestling on mats, crawling their way through the brightly colored play tunnel. Guests had congregated, a few of my friends grouping off to commiserate with one another, Diana's people from Narcotics Anonymous nursing cups of punch, talking with her friends from graduate school, everyone stunned, staring at one another, trying to figure out what to say. Diana had been through chemo, radiation, two bone marrow transplants, all for what? I remember a pair of long-arguing lovers making out in my sister's closet.

As if propelled from a cannon, Lily left me and Susannah and Crystal and her grandma behind, bursting toward the heart of the party. Some of her zags had to be pent-up energy: anywhere she looked brought someone she knew, a loved adult, another child she wanted to play with. Of course, logic suggests she was searching for one person in particular.

THE NEXT MORNING, I watched Lily, splayed out on Mommy's side of the bed, where she and Diana had always slept, entwined. The top of Lily's head peeked out from beneath the comforter, her hairline was high on her skull. Hair—dirty brown, thin, and unkempt—was damp, curled in places from how she slept.

As soon as Lily woke, I began.

"Listen to me."

My therapist, Dr. Mark Roberts, had provided the script. He was primarily a couples therapist. Diana and I had started seeing him during her pregnancy. After she fell ill, I just kept going, alone.

I stayed up late into the night, rehearsing these sentences, verbatim, into the bathroom mirror:

"Your mother is in heaven," I said.

Lily was following along.

"She was very sick and had to go away."

I kept eye contact.

"She loves you very much. Your mom wanted to be here with you. She tried very hard to be here for you. We all tried as hard as we could. Your mom still loves you, Lily. She will always love you. She will always be in your heart just like you will always be in her heart."

My daughter's eyes are unnaturally large, and give her face a particularly moonlike quality. For the rest of my days I'll be tortured by how, in these moments, those eyes grew.

"Mommy's gone? Where's Mommy? When is she coming back?"

WHEN THAT LITTLE purplish body slipped into this world, I made sure to keep my own eyes focused: I felt devotion, felt what I imagine to be the requisite amount of awe. Still, the newborn had not gestated inside me. Mine was not the breast Lily would feed at. I hadn't suffered eighteen hours of labor without an epidural. Nor had I experienced being stretched open. I surely hadn't gone through any of that legendary, primordial, mystic maternal bonding. There was a limit to how involved I could be. Plus, your early infant is unformed, not possessing a specific personality so much as pile of traits—colicky, tearful, sleepy, placid. Honestly, even as those nascent characteristics had begun their formulation, as Lily's habits started to build, my brain still was wrapping itself around the fact that I even *was* a dad. Diana absorbed every change to her baby child, little miracle girl, as a cosmic wonder. Me? I was concerned about logistics, irritated when I had to exchange the diapers I'd just bought from CVS, because it was time to get the larger size. Still, I handled my business. I stayed up through my designated midnight-to-dawn shifts, cuddling our baby, entertaining myself with goo-goo talk. *"You don't know what I'm saying, do you? No, you have no idea."* I strapped on the baby carrier and hauled Lily to the park, giving her mom a chance to shower or nap. *"All right, let's get trucking, little trucker."* On the regular, I got down on my knees, fumbled with our portable changing station. With the correct Huggies ready, I dove into the stink and muck, occasionally looking up, staring into her sparkling, innocent eyes, crooning the little ditty I'd made up for these occasions:

> Diaper Change
> It's time for Diaper Change
> There's something very strange
> Below the mountain range!

DECEMBER 19. ELEVEN days after Diana passed. Eight days after Lily's third birthday. Holiday season heading into overdrive, most everyone we knew had hightailed it out of town. The little one and I faced a long stretch with just the two of us, together—no sitters, not a lot of help—in the frigid and tourist-packed city. It was daunting, sure, but dinner had been painless and unmemorable, and I felt good about the day just behind us, and the fun part of the night about to start. In half an hour, we'd Skype with Peg back in Memphis. Then it would be jammies, brushing her teeth, washing her face, all the rituals of winding down, easing into bedtime.

One way of killing time and tiring her out involved races down the carpeted hallway just outside our apartment. Lily loved sprints, the long hallways, and she especially lit up when I'd disappear, hide in the stairwell, and surprise her. Tonight, for no discernible reason, Lily sprinted into the elevator. We ended up racing down the marble floor in the building's lobby. I was in my socks, which was against our rules for hallway running, but the game would only take a few minutes, so big whoop. Lily sped right out of the elevator door— *game on!* I caught up and passed her, stepping up my pace, actually running kind of fast. An idea flashed; it seemed surprising, the kind of jolt that would entertain Lily: I transitioned into a version of the standing slide that, back in his first starring role, helped make young Tom Cruise a teen heartthrob. Unlike Tom, I had pants on. Also unlike him, I kept on sliding. It was fun at first. Except I possessed so much momentum that my feet went out from under me, and zoomed right over my head.

The impact was shocking, a wall of force through my lower back. For seconds afterward I couldn't believe how much it hurt.

Glee in her face, Lily started laughing. *Daddy and his funny pratfalls.* There's little better on earth than bringing joy into your toddler's face. But in this moment her laugh struck me, this detail off in a way that might have been ominous.

I'd landed near the Christmas tree our management company always put out for the season. Hanging from one of the lower branches was an ornament, this red ball Lily had convinced me to purchase a few days earlier, at a stand on Second Avenue.

I must have put my arm down to cushion the impact, because just below my right elbow swelling had started: a knot already the size of a lemon.

I tried to get to my feet, but when I pressed down—putting pressure on my right foot, trying to push upward—white-hot pain ran through my right side. Blinding pain.

Lily's face changed. She looked worried, ready to cry.

"It's fine," I told her.

Silence through the lobby. No one coming or going.

Lily kept waiting, kept watching me, those huge, frying pan eyes desperate, like always, to take in every single possible detail.

THERE'S A LONG section in *The Wind-Up Bird Chronicle* by Haruki Murakami in which a man is forced to jump down a well. The well is impossibly deep. When the man lands, the impact shatters bones in his leg. There is no light down there. The stone around him is impossible to climb. No food. Some morning dew he can lick off the stones, but not enough to survive on. He feels around and comes across the bones of all the poor animals that have fallen down this well over the years. The nightmare of all nightmares. You could not possibly be more fucked than he is. Murakami allowed this man to escape because his fiction doesn't abide by the physical laws of our reality.

Reader, I was stuck inside the physical laws of our reality. According to these laws, I was forty-two, a recent widower, deeply grieving. I had no full-time job, no investments, no retirement account, barely a dented pot to piss in. Until recently, I'd been one of those fathers who sometimes, despite himself, referred to his infant as "it." Flat on my back in the lobby of our apartment building, it sure looked like

I'd just destroyed half of my body in a freak accident, with my right elbow shattered and useless, and some kind of break—Jesus, I hoped it wasn't a break—through my hip. And I was solely and wholly responsible for the care, feeding, and well-being of this recently motherless, blameless little girl.

If it was possible to be under the bottom of the well, that's where I was. Where *we* were. Fucked. We were deeply and irrevocably fucked.

This is the starting point.

CHAPTER TWO

Regardless of what happens in the world, I'm still going to do the same thing every day, which is to Love, Serve, Remember, Love, Serve, Remember. Whatever you need to do to get ready to die, you should have done it a minute ago. Or do it now and get ready. Every minute is the minute in which you die again. A conscious being is holding on nowhere.
                                —Diana Colbert, note to self, 2010

DIANA AND I met at a mutual friend's party in Williamsburg, Brooklyn, just as that neighborhood was getting gentrified. The woman throwing the party wanted us to meet, actually, and made a point of introducing us. Diana: this pale and freckled and curvy lady in formfitting leather pants. A bit of her midriff visible, spilling over. Streaks of blond amid thick brown hair that fell down to her shoulders. Oddly open face. I am six feet tall, and she looked at me square, maintaining eye contact as I worked my particular brand of charm on her, meaning that she bore with me as I mansplained the difference between two prog-rock bands that, to be honest, have little difference between them. Diana's eyes were big and trusting. She handed me one of the business cards she'd just had printed up. The cards represented her move to get clients as a massage therapist, which, she explained, would allow her to quit being a receptionist. We stayed side by side, talking, until she told me she had another friend's party to attend that night. I volunteered to tag along. She did not drink at either function. Neither did I.

No irony to her. Even less guile. But a stellar listener: what you had to say was part of that larger vibe she gave off; how you were doing mattered to her. Once, I found a note she wrote to herself. It worked out the importance of "wishing for others to be happy, but also endeavoring toward unlimited, unconditional friendliness toward oneself, which then naturally radiates outward to others." That twisting message, I think, captures a part of her: a probing, new-agey, people-pleasing aspect, yes, but also an intelligence. This intelligence was deep, it was intricate, although, oftentimes, people who conducted themselves in a manner that one might consider urbane (or *shrewd*) used her good nature, the ease with which she might agree, or give someone the benefit of the doubt, as an excuse to ignore her, dismiss her, or just take her for granted. I saw this happen. Early in our dating life, I did it myself. One afternoon, we left her Prospect Place apartment, and were halfway down the street when she stopped and hugged a tree.

"What the hell?" I asked.

Answer. "Oh, I just like to hug this tree. I don't know. It brings me comfort."

I likely made a face. My mind started: How much of the tree hugging was performative, done to show herself as eccentric? How much did she want to show herself as heartfelt?

What was undeniable: every day she hauled her heavy-ass massage table—twenty pounds? thirty?—on her back and went on the subway from Brooklyn to Manhattan and her private clients. Diana also worked at spas on weekends. She'd borrowed the money for massage school from her stepmother and was determined to pay back every cent. She was less determined about the money she owed to NYU for an education she'd compromised by rolling too many blunts. Once, she wrote a grant proposal asking for money so she could give massages to homeless people with AIDS; when she didn't get the money, she gave them the massages anyway. After too many men wanted a different type of massage, the sessions ceased. On our first date, I picked her up after her twelve-step meeting. One of her diets had her counting out Fritos. She'd also walk a mile uphill, into the wind, neck-deep in snow, if at the end of the trek, there was a slice of key lime pie.

An only child. A child of divorce. A polite Southern girl. She'd adored the cousins she'd grown up with in suburban Memphis; some of her happiest times had been spent in her aunt and uncle's house when all the relatives were over and celebrating Thanksgiving. That was the joyous environment she'd idealized: a full house of raucous children. It was what she'd wanted more than anything. To be a mother.

THE MALE'S CAPACITY to feel sorry for himself is bottomless: once you take that first step, it's an easy slide down. It is no lie when I tell you that, after my accident in the apartment building lobby, I was a downhill champion.

Four days in a dark hospital ward with a television playing somewhere outside of my field of vision. Bedpans galore. Reconstructive surgery on my elbow, screws holding everything together, bones set and reset, my right arm immobile in a soft cast. Also, the hairline fracture across my hip, meaning I'd spend a month laid up, but also that if I moved around too much during that month, and the fracture deepened into a break, I'd be out of commission for half a year. Obviously, the threat loomed. To try and help, the industrious folks at Bellevue Hospital—bless them each and every one—rigged up a specialized, double-decker walker. It was a monstrosity: imagine monkey bars, or maybe construction scaffolding, reaching up to your chest. I had to put all my weight on its bars instead of my arm or hip, so just getting from my desk across my small living room meant lurching around on it, looking like some kind of fifties movie monster.

None of it was fun, but I managed to lurch my way out of Bellevue, back to my longtime apartment on Twenty-Second, the home base Lily knew. Almost immediately I was presented with a brand-new ordeal. If I so much as looked at the lamp on my bureau, I was transported, suddenly in New Orleans just after Katrina, when Diana and I had built houses with Habitat for Humanity—sitting together on a carved bench in a small antique shop, needing to check out of our room and get to the airport, we'd waited for that lamp to get bubble wrapped.

If I opened a drawer, if I looked on a counter—if any random object came into my line of vision—some version of this memory hole opened: a deck of cards connected me to poker nights in Memphis with Diana's family; a Buddhist tchotchke reminded me, for whatever reason, of the time my Shih Tzu went missing and Diana had paid for a phone session with a pet psychic, and how, when I heard this news, I got confused and a little mad, and then suddenly I also had my long-overdue realization; finally, I'd understood: her tree hugging had been heartfelt.

WE HAD A decade together, courtship and marriage. Our one serious disagreement had been about having a kid. I refused to do it. I needed to finish my book first. No negotiating on this. I'd been banging on my pipe dream of a novel since the tail end of my twenties, eating massive loads of shit along the way. Third-shift legal proofreader, tabloid rewrite guy, ghostwriter, filcher of reams of typing paper from office supply closets—that was me. I was that long-haired dude who was too old to be hoarding chicken wings from the cater-waiter tray, who'd fielded a *decade* of six in the morning calls from my mom about when I was going to apply to law school. Even my best friends assumed I'd never finish the thing. Maybe Diana didn't believe, either, but too bad: she'd chosen her horse and so got dragged along for the ride. This meant sitting on her ovaries through what turned into the heart of her thirties, including one nine-month stretch when I made like the drummer from an eighties Sunset Strip band and charged our groceries to her credit card. Waiting also meant she put together a DIY wedding for a whopping seven grand, that she voluntarily took classes and converted to Judaism just so my mom would be happy at the wedding, that she came up with a honeymoon where we basically drove around Vermont in an old Volvo, stopping at roadside vistas and feeding each other the last layer of our wedding cake (buttercream icing, fluffy chocolate sponge; it was the best, *the best*). And, too, Diana recognized that her body could only take so much of the grind of being a massage therapist. She realized that she wanted to go back to school, then nailed the grad school tests. Earning a scholarship, she pursued a master's at UMass Amherst in the literature of nineteenth-century colonialism, our first married year passing with us in different states, juggling a long-distance relationship. All that and finally, finally, *finally*, I finished my book. Got the damn thing actually published.

And I *still* put her off.

BOTTOM LINE: YOU can't tell the woman you are sharing this life with that she cannot have your child. I couldn't, anyway. So, yes, add me to the bazillions of men stunned and dragged into the yoke of fatherhood. Although, really, what was I avoiding? Handling my share of the bills, okay, you kind of have to do that. Hitching up the baby sling every now and then. Some good tickle fights. A lot of nodding sagely to friends, explaining that, as good progressive partners, "we're co-parenting."

But I was not happy about the situation we were in. I wasn't tricked into the pregnancy, but I felt tricked *by* it. *Technically, I have a kid now,* I thought. *But oh well.* I'd eaten so much crap in pursuit of becoming a writer, now that I was a published novelist, I wanted to do all the cool published-novelist stuff. I had never been to Europe. I wanted us to go. I wanted to see the world. Diana wanted to be a mom? Let her. I remained determined to make up for lost time from my career, to sink my canines into literary success's fleshy hind parts, go hard after magazine assignments, pitch screenplays, write operas in space, just basically burn burn burn all of those fabulous yellow roman candles from Kerouac which explode in mixed metaphors on five ends.

That had been my mindset. My wife wanted to be a mom? Great: I was along for the ride.

DIANA WAS DIAGNOSED with leukemia when Lily was six months old. Checking on what we both assumed was a flu, she learned that her white blood cell count was dangerously low, that cancer was the probable diagnosis. The doctors pushed to hospitalize her immediately, ordered an ambulance to transport her, two hours, to a research hospital. Diana wanted to check herself out of that ER right there, take herself and the baby straight to a Buddhist monastery. Lily was with us in the exam room, playing with a plastic glove that had been blown up into a five-fingered balloon. Diana and I looked at one another, no clue, nowhere to begin, certainly no answers other than the largest answer: that is, the answer that emerged in how we looked at one another. Despite or maybe in lieu of the terror of the situation, our bodies involuntarily gravitated toward each other. Our petty grudges, our growing disagreements, all the fissures and log-gerheads that were emerging in our marriage—they gave way. From diagnosis on, I devoted myself to the health of my ill wife, the care of our baby daughter. And Diana surrendered to the wishes of her many loved ones—and, yes, that's me waving at the front of the line. She did *not* go into a monastery and meditate away the cancer. Instead, she gave herself to science, and to what extended, step by miserable step, into a two-and-a-half-year marathon: more chemotherapy than any sane person could imagine; enough radiation to make her body visible from Jupiter; weeks at a time beneath a futuristic, medical breathing tent; all that *plus* two full bone marrow transplants. She let her physical self be attacked and diminished. I'd like to say it was so the two of us freaks could grow old and soft together. Maybe that was part of it. But there was another reason, one far more important, playing with that five-fingered balloon.

THREE YEARS OLD now, that little reason, and fearless, determined to go down the big kids' slide, reach up toward the monkey bars. Second week of January—one month after the accident. Unseason-ably tepid, sun starting to set. She was over by the swings, springing forward, sticking out her chin, clamping down on her jaw, clomping those unsteady toddler clomps, that impossible spring to her step. Little hell on tiny wheels, only not wheels: pink sneakers that lit up in the soles, coordinated with one of those taffeta princess skirts, the outline of her Pull-Ups diaper ballooning from the back of her tights (thick pink stripes). Lily Starr Colbert-Bock, Silly Lily, Señorita Lilisita Mon Amita. On cue her voice, high, girly, her toddler flub of words, her cute breaking laughter: "*Watch me, Daddy!*" she called from across the playground, and of course followed up with an epic face-plant, after which came her ambulance siren screams, which faded as suddenly as they'd arrived. A shameless flirter. A true charmer. Once in a while shy with new people, especially if she liked or felt curious about them, but mostly open, those wide gray eyes fixing on you, inviting: *Dive in, the water's perfect.*

Back at the apartment, me on the couch, the Tomato Tornado below, bent at the waist, tracking a stray orange pacifier. Calling each pacifier she chews her *da-doo*, she picked that da-doo right off the carpet and put it in her mouth and I did not stop her because I am lazy. One of those teething deals, the way she still goes to town on da-doos, but also part of a bigger oral fixation—likely rooted in having to stop breastfeeding early, moving to formula and bottle at six months, when her mom had chemo. Her fixation also might have had something to do with how she used to gnaw on spoons, how much she still adores lollipops, although what child of three does not want a lollipop? Does not want a cookie? Lily, Destroyer of Pizzas! Epic mess maker! Tonight she had ice cream on her cheeks, her chin, her blouse, whatever else you got, ice cream's there, too! Would not so much as try carrots at dinner, but sometimes willing to give pad Thai a shot, and brussels sprouts, and broccoli. A pretty good little eater, actually, though I still have to be careful: strawberries and raspberries sometimes give her a rash. Wait, how did she get ahold of that roll of twine? What could I have been thinking to leave twine within her arm's reach? Goddamn twine. All over the living room, beneath the couch. "*How?*" I asked.

Her response: an inquisitive, almost gentle look. C*ould there possibly be a problem with the destruction I have wrought?* Petal lips form other questions she did not ask. Her hair starting to go long in back but oftentimes did not hold the braid. Shockingly good at logic and memory games. Loved tea parties with her tea party plates. And stickers, hot damn she *loved* stickers, placing them on toy cups, on my desks, on walls—everywhere—sparkly stickers, especially. My girl. My girl. Getting her face painted was heaven. Stuffed animals were her jam. Baths were particularly joyous, too, at the end of the evening, a way to get the ice cream and flecks of twine off her cheeks, a means of holding night-night at bay, sure, but also in-the-moment rapture. Loved bubbles. Adored the little green octopus bath toy when the lights at the end of each green arm went bright. And the splashing. Splashing made her howl with laughter—again, that wonderful, high-pitched, fully committed, little-girl soul laugh. Who could get enough of that laugh? Glowed the sweat of angels. Baby smell remaining on her even while she soaked. Inordinately patient afterward while I put on her jammies. Patient in a way that seemed almost delicate toward me, understanding that Daddy was getting better, it still took Daddy a bit.

TACKED TO THE door of our lone bedroom's closet was a screen print. It took up around the top half of the door, so figure about three feet tall, maybe half as wide. Originally commissioned as merch for an indie band (the Phenomenauts) appearing at a San Francisco venue. An ogre. Radioactive green. Ripped with muscles. Wearing a spiked motorcycle helmet and dragging his knuckles along the surface of the moon. His ogre grin was wide, toothy, and drooling at its corners. Perched on his ogre shoulder was a pixie in a metallic pink spacesuit; within her glittering, fishbowl helmet, she smiled.

Ogre Shouldering Pixie was aspirational for me, a model for who I *could* be.

The night particularly frigid. Beneath the rock poster's purview, Lily and I began our bedtime ritual, getting comfy under the covers.

When Mom had been sick, we'd all slept in the bed together. Now it was me and Lily, with Lily claiming Mommy's side.

My arm, in its soft cast, had limited mobility. I fumbled to hold the storybook, one of my favorites to read to her, the adventure of a lion who wanders into a library.

Doing as Daddy said, being careful of my cast, she curled herself into my side, a little package, getting in the best angled position for some good cuddles. The top of her head rubbed against my chin. She played with my facial hair, nuzzled into my neck.

For my part, I leaned into her; as I did, her breath arrived on my face—faint, hot bursts scented with the remnants of dinner, whiffs her toothpaste had not blocked out.

"I want to start with *Angelina Ballerina*," Lily said.

I put down the story I actually liked and rummaged through the bedside picture books. Okay. The narcissist mouse who wants to be a prima ballerina.

When that was done, Lily ordered: "Amos and Bobo."

"Right," I said. "*Amos & Boris*."

The adventurous mouse who builds a boat but is puny, so he gets carried along by an ocean wave, then is rescued by the kind whale.

Lily wasn't sleepy. "More."

Final story. A gorilla who lets animals, one by one, out of their cages, leads them out of the zoo. Before I turned each cardboard page, I pointed out, in that picture, the same little rodent, always bringing up the rear. With much glee, Lily and I exclaimed, our voices overlapping: "Mouse with banana!"

Tonight, four fingers—tiny and soft and delicate—attached themselves, hooking around my right thumb, the thumb sticking out of my soft cast.

Those little fingers curling caught me. Their light grip made me pause.

It was a lightning strike. I was stricken.

An instantaneous recalibration, untold switches within me turning red to green, my lungs opening, clean breaths entering, my world expanding.

My father, while he drove, used to reach out with his off hand, toward me in the back seat, wanting a quick slapped five, a clasp of fingers, some kind of dap. When was the first time that, of my own volition, I grasped his hand like that? I would have been Lily's age. Maybe in our dirt backyard? As a child I loved him reaching out for me, even when he improvised, turning his hand into a villain trying to eat me up. The teenaged me wanted to be my own person, took his reaching to be a sign of weakness, and turned into a cold fish, limply acquiescing, desiring to break free.

A friend of mine named Sean believes there is no way to understand your parents until you become a parent.

In our bed, instantly, I understood—at least, my daughter taking my hand, believing in me.

ONCE STORY TIME was finished, I shut off the lamp on the bedside table, broke out my laptop. "Hooray," Lily said. She wiggled, adjusted herself, used my chest as a viewing platform. Each night ended for us this way, with YouTube: first, *Sesame Street* fare—the pop singer Feist, who rhymed "*one two three four*" with "*chickens just back from the shore.*" A friend had once told me "Musicals are love," and this was a message I'd taken to heart. So we also watched various timeless sequences, clips from *Singin' in the Rain, Annie, Mary Poppins, The Sound of Music.*

The Von Trapps concluded. I tried to calm Lily's jangly body. My voice soft, I attempted, without success, to stay in tune:

"Jeremiah was a bullfrog . . ."

MAYBE A MINUTE after her birth, the very first time I held Lily: her full body not even running the length of my forearm. I was in shock, marveling at her tiny form, her wrinkled face purple with blood. And I sang to her. The same song I sang right now, that I'd sing every night to her.

After "Joy to the World," I sang the song whose guitar solo had blared out of speakers in the rolling green field, right after Diana and I had wed: "Sweet Child O' Mine."

Tonight, on Twenty-Second Street, she'd taken my hand, reaffirmed her grip on my heart; I stared at the fluorescent stars glued to our ceiling, continued adoring my daughter, waited for her to yawn, to stop twitching.

I lay there and couldn't help myself, thinking of Diana's last year on this earth. She hadn't been healthy enough to walk around a city block. To get in and out of our apartment building, we'd needed a wheelchair and a special ramp.

Toward the end, her ample five-foot-ten frame a wasted stalk, just a hundred or so pounds. The hair that had grown in after her last bone marrow transplant was falling out, her front teeth going dark in a way that couldn't have been healthy. She was ensconced in her fuzzy robe with the ducks. Once-strong hands, now frail, clutched our little pudge ball. Beneath some extra blankets, they were both strapped into the wheelchair. Diana's faculties had to be compromised, but she was still ordering me, "*Careful.*" Lily, meanwhile, remained entranced, clapping, giggling.

From the moment Diana had become ill, she'd told Lily, "Mommy is in your heart and you are in Mommy's heart." Even in the midst of our hell, we had these moments when Lily was energized with her mother's joy. Diana's middle name was Joy.

After what that woman had been through, after how she'd fought, I couldn't blame her for not being here.

Which didn't prevent the bedroom's empty dark space from expanding around me, from closing in on me, both at the same time.

I also thought about Peg, Lily's grandma.

And Susannah, Lily's godmother.

Mommy's in your heart. You are in Mommy's heart.

Could Diana be looking out for Lily through the hearts of the people who loved her?

I closed my hand around Lily's—barely a hand, so tiny, at three.

And recalled my own hand, so safe inside my father's.

A cynic, which I like to pretend I am, might claim I was in love with my memories, enraptured by this look back into my own youth. Sure. Who isn't?

But this chain of time and love felt so profound to me. It seemed I might actually be able to raise her.

Simultaneously, a terror arrived through the chambers of my heart, many gongs pounding:

If Diana was going to be taking care of Lily, at the end of the day, the heavy lifting would be through me.

It had to be through me.

YET THE QUESTION remained. *How?*

Nobody put Daddy Warbucks and Daddy Von Trapp and Cinderella Daddy in absolute either/or dynamics, demanding they give up their manhood, surrender their livelihood, be round-the-clock responsible for their kids' daily bathing habits, homeschooling, social lives, wardrobes, the whole matzo ball. Nonetheless, each man was presented with the opportunity to seriously show up, to engage—deeply, at the foundational level—in the emotional and physical development of their young children. These men had the chance to be present, to care, and to experience—profoundly so—the natural outgrowth of all that care. They had the chance to create true emotional intimacy with their kids during foundational stretches of childhood. That's a big deal. Instead, they outsourced.

Truth is, our home was no stranger to sitters. When Diana was sick, having Lily around may have nourished her soul, but there was no way she could physically look after the kid. Taking Lily to indoor areas with other children wasn't an option, as it meant the risk of Lily bringing home germs to Diana, who basically had no immune system. Our toddler could not sit still for three literal seconds, but wasn't able to go to day care, couldn't attend story time at a library, wasn't even allowed to run with and touch other children at playgrounds. Our solution involved setting fire to part of our meager savings, hiring shifts of young women. Ko, a Vietnamese student in her early twenties, became a mainstay, doing yeoman's work through Diana's final month, occupying Lily's days with trips to museums, and venturing to restaurants deep in Brooklyn, where Ko's friends worked. (During down moments after the lunch rush, they taught Lily how to use chopsticks.)

As I healed from my accident, I kept relying on Ko; after a few weeks, she stopped showing up, blew off my texts.

I interviewed an alumnus from my grad school. Dyed hair, nose ring, teeming with good energy, she seemed like a perfect part-time nanny.

First afternoon on the job, she started slurring, slouched on the couch—a total heroin nod. She managed to drag herself back into consciousness, rose, and staggered out the front door, never to return.

The network of friends who'd helped during Diana's illness had stopped calling and coming over, receding back into their lives.

Understandable; there were limits to how much time people could give, right? Reader, when I asked for help, my in-box filled with referrals. Contact info. Gushing emails. The bubbly junior publicist with golden tresses and extensive babysitting experience; the charming daughter who was home after college and between jobs: Lindsey, Lauren, Liza, even names that did not begin with *L*. Always in their early twenties. Broke as shit. Scraping together a side hustle. *Willing to potentially babysit weekends. Might be able to work a few nights a week, until internship.*

Laid out on the sofa bed that Diana and I had purchased at a thrift store whose proceeds went to fighting AIDS, I kept dribbling my basketball against the glazed brick wall, thereby increasing my hand strength, dexterity, and coordination.

Laid out on my late wife's yoga mat, talking on my landline, I negotiated with the banking rep who steadfastly refused—no matter how much documentation I sent—to transfer the remaining money from Diana's account into one set up in Lily's name.

Sitting in the ergonomic rolling chair I'd purchased for myself from a fancy catalogue right after I'd sold the book, I kept my Nokia perched against my ear and listened. My sister Crystal continued her role as my lifelong best friend and buoy. She let me know she was still unearthing clothes from Lily's stay during my hospital ordeal, planned on bringing everything over as soon as she found a spot in her schedule. Crystal had a young son almost Lily's age, was pregnant to boot. She nonetheless asked if she could pick up anything special that I or the little cannoli might like. Then, in her unique, supportive, and thoroughly no-bullshit way, Crystal flipped a switch, dispensed with the preliminaries, and started laying down the law, informing me that Manhattan day care was no joke and I had to get off my ass and fill out those applications. And I'd better ask friends for those letters of recommendation. And it did not matter if the fall was nine months away, Charles. She knew I was grieving. But she was on my side here. So, please, I had to not be a dick. Just take care of this.

I mumbled assurances.

I watched the next sitter, Michele, overcome the introductory burst of shyness that served as my daughter's opening gambit.

I watched the sitter after that. Kneeling down on our living room rug (nicknamed "the snow rug throw rug"), she learned about the adventures of a stuffed animal, in the process winning Lily's confidence.

Lily let these young women put her hair in ponytails and clips.

Let them put food into her mouth.

Let them bathe her and towel her off.

She engaged with them, learned how to be coy with them, how to charm them. She followed their leads, repeated their phrases, absorbed their mannerisms.

Lauren bartered with her (follow enough instructions, Lily got a lollipop); Liza always took her to the CVS (for nail polish? a glittery headband?). When Lindsey came around, Lily asked, "We go to Baskin-Robbins?" Lindsey made her promise: afterwards, she'd brush brushy brush her teeth.

Corralling those golden tresses into her knit cap, Lindsey confirmed the dates of her next visit, slipped the check into her coat pocket. "Okay, I'm leaving." Her voice was purposefully theatrical. "Anybody want to say goodbye?"

Sitting at the little white table that served as her desk and meal area, Lily made a point of concentrating on her drawing. A singsong response: "No, I don't."

"All right, see you later!"

In the hallway, they'd hug. Before that, however, as per their ritual, Lindsey had to open our front door. And when this happened, Lily turned desperate. Arms pumping, running as hard as she could, Lily had to give chase. Before the young woman left, Lily had to catch her.

SCOTT FITZGERALD FAMOUSLY intoned that plot is character. His reasoning was that the situation a character finds themselves in always ends up an outgrowth of who he or she is. Looking back, I see that I was an overgrown, adult child myself.

I write this ten years after the fact. From such distance, I can see how I wanted to have it both ways: to make sure Lily was cared for and happy, yes, but at the same time to continue to basically sweep in on the weekends and tickle, doing the minimum, or the near minimum, so as to stay inside my pillowy bubble of creative, arrested development, claiming I was taking care of the kid when actually I was *avoiding* the true work of parenting. *Terrified of it.*

I did not want to do this. I did not want to raise this child.

But the die had been rolled. Such was my task. Such was my journey. And whether or not I loved my daughter (most def); whether I'd taken responsibility for her of my own free will (certainly I had not); whether I was setting out on this lifelong journey by choice (also no); whether I was mentally prepared for or capable of what I was undertaking (good one); whether I was mature enough, had the discipline required, the necessary self-awareness, the abilities for reflection, adaptation; whether I could cede my ego and petty desires; whether I would sabotage myself, come up short, lash out, self-destruct, and /or try to quit—none of these questions mattered; at the very least, they were less significant than the raw truth, the larger happening, this journey already underway.

Our ramshackle love story was already unfolding. This was going to define me.

Was I up to the challenge?

My little girl had returned from the hallway. She was by my side, reaching for my hand, a pink pixie wanting to perch herself on the green ogre's shoulder.

Fuck.

CHAPTER THREE

STUDIES SHOW THAT losing one's mother during an early age is likely to do long-term damage to a child's self-esteem, to her capacity to express feelings and to trust. The younger the kid is when she loses her mother, the more likely she is to develop anxiety and behavioral issues, as well as problems with drugs and alcohol. Girls who lose their mothers are more likely to become sexually active earlier in life. They are more likely to have difficulties maintaining relationships as adults, and they tend to develop an unconscious fear of intimacy.

So then, like, what if the girl isn't properly taught by her father to look both ways before crossing the street, and on a snowy day is eager to get to the park with her sled, and she runs into traffic, all while her dad is busy reading a text with yet another round of edits for a freelance piece that he needs done, as he needs that check to clear?

What about . . . if Dad reminds her to wear her scarf but forgets to say one word about her gloves, and she goes out and keeps her hands in her pockets to avoid freezing, but it's still too cold outside, and she gets frostbite and loses the top of her right thumb?

If she grows up thinking pizza is health food?

If she doesn't learn to clean up after herself, doesn't know how to make her bed, can't put on a fitted sheet?

If she gets the date wrong, forgets to carry the number into the next column?

If she leaps from seeking the approval of her dad to needing the approval of some dreamy guy from the junior college and is knocked up before she's sixteen?

If she doesn't learn how to go along to get along? If she is like her dad and doesn't have an internal filter and constantly says the wrong thing? If she can't listen, can't hear what's really being said to her?

If she does not understand or employ traditional feminine wiles that, offensive though it may be to admit, are necessary to getting along in a patriarchy? If she cannot use flattery and flirtation as tools—to entice, to defuse, to protect and promote herself?

Or, conversely, if she does not have confidence in her intelligence? If she doesn't know when to speak up? If she is defensive, secretive, paranoid, unable to trust, unable to love?

If she makes bad deals, hurries into lopsided partnerships, capsizes friendships, torches important relationships? If she fucks up and fucks up and keeps on fucking things up?

I couldn't think this way.

FOR NOW, ALL hail the ass end of winter! Praise be its therapeutic powers! Soft cast *falling away*. Right arm *mostly functional*. Right hip *still diminished, but stronger*, no longer in need of that contraption; my body *actually kinda sorta working!*

Similarly transformed was the cluttered world of our apartment—I mean, yes, it was every bit as overstuffed; there was little to zero light in the living room and bedroom; the kitchen remained a kitchenette, just one person at a time could use it. The great majority of the place's walls continued to be thin as rice paper, only now the rice paper walls were bright with primary colors. Cardboard posters that had scribbly Magic Marker drawings tacked to them; a chalk-board with positive sayings; charts with completed tasks translating into shiny stars—in short, any image that could make our home look cheery and bright, as opposed to a ship's hold at midnight. Huge swaths of my first novel had been written down in the bottom of this dark hold, with me listening to late-night sports talk radio; now I kept a midnight bedtime rule (okay, sometimes I stretched it to one), so I'd be fresh in the morning for the little girl. Similar reasoning meant sayonara to my usual four-day scruff of facial hair, to my Buddhist beads that weren't around my wrist for reasons of peace and love but because they looked like a bunch of skulls, to my T-shirts celebrating the baroque and hard rocking and sexually pro-vocative. Instead, this child would know her father as clean-shaven, put together, reasonably neat, someone who wiped his lenses clean on the regular, who was not at all beneath the bottom of a well.

Almost noon. Here's Lily in her pink Hello Kitty jammies, want-ing to know: "Why do forks have sticks at the end?"

I had been cutting construction paper. I put down the scissors. Using my hand like a broom, I swept up and gathered, from my desk, all these newly formed creations, triangles made of colored pieces of cardboard. "Because space aliens can't get spaghetti to stick to their tentacles, duh."

Dumping my misshapen triangles, I spread them, random falling constellations, over the snow rug throw rug, and thus prepared our newest time-wasting activity.

"Okay," I said. "New game."

Lily clapped. Soon enough, we were balancing on our toes, step-ping carefully, avoiding all colored pieces.

"Don't step on the stinky cheese," Lily cackled.

"Step on the stinky cheese," I warned, "you will get a *BLUMPO*."

"A *BLUMPO*?" More cackling. "What's a *BLUMPO*?"

Blum•po. *Noun*. 1. The penalty for stepping on a fictional slice of stinky cheese. 2. A disruption, whether in the progress of a game or to the joyous nature of an outing. 3. Disagreement, irritation.

How about that collection of gingerbread houses—each one inspired by a New York City landmark—that were on display at the fancy midtown hotel where we ate at the secret hamburger stand? Was that a blumpo?

How about the Brooklyn food trucks we visited? The pop-up temporary tattoo parlor?

Outside of Lincoln Center before the start of the circus, she'd balanced on the lip of the fountains and stretched her poofy-coated arms out wide to the world, and just then the water sprayed out above her and she lit up—amazed, joyous. Did that qualify, was that one of those nefarious blumpos?

Was one found inside the iconic Plaza Hotel, where Eloise inspired chaos? (Lily and I had tea, left the requisite postcard for everyone's favorite long-term guest.)

Standing on line with me to get into the Lego store in Rockefeller Center. Standing on line with me to ride the carousel under the Brooklyn Bridge. Standing on line with me for the Chelsea Piers carousel. For the carousel at Bryant Park. On line with me at the Fourteenth Street Foot Locker for a re-release of the White Cement Jordan 3s I'd salivated over as a college freshman but never owned.

Truth: I needed places for us to go, classes to take, things for us to do. I lived in terror—mortal terror—of empty afternoons, their procession of minutes without end. How much time could we really burn tiptoeing around cut-out triangles? With a few rounds of memory card games? How much time learning that yellow and blue make green? With simple arithmetic on the laptop and the site's background music numbing my mind like so much novocaine?

When I was a teenager trying to play basketball, and our team was getting blown out, Coach Mangold used to set incremental goals as a way of getting our squad back into the game: "Let's cut it to sixteen, let's get it to ten by halftime." In my case, this became its own plan: *At ten on Saturday we'll go to the overpriced new retro diner. Then she can play with the Groovy Girls dolls at Barnes & Noble. After nappy time, maybe we hit the math museum.*

We did them all. They were exhausting. They worked my patience, frayed my nerves.

Not one was a blumpo.

Even better, for Lily, than all these forays: the chance to share and bond with children her age. YMCA day camp.

The final day, I arrived to find Lily waiting for me, her face especially bright.

Not only had she enjoyed a *fifth* full day of play; today also had given her cause to feel singularly proud. A week of all those other kids taking trips to the bathroom with the counselors had provided the impetus; she had been able to implement all our prep work and urging ("Pushie with your tushie") and had scooted over the rim of that physical and olfactory milestone. Our diaper-change song was no longer necessary. A sacrifice, but one that both of us were proud to make. She beamed: "I did it."

And so there we were, me and my wondrous Tomato Tornado, busting serious ass—at least, as much as my rusty right hip allowed. We were heading east on Fourteenth, returning home, triumphant and celebratory, from the Y. Lily was safely strapped into the seat of our lightweight, but trustworthy Maclaren stroller. Gifted to me by my mom and sis, its rain-resistant fabric was the bright yellow of Big Bird, the yellow of streaming, golden sunlight.

Lily was sort of reclining and looking comfortable, her legs akimbo, her knees pointing in opposite directions. Half sucking her thumb, her eyes glossy, she appeared, in this moment, to be one extremely satiated princess, zoning out until her next entertainment appeared.

Behind her, I was pushing like hell. You can see me: six feet tall or thereabouts, thin but with a bit of a middle from stress snacking, this grown-ass man with *Peppa Pig* stickers on the shoulder of his monstrous winter coat. I was giving a heads-up to that elderly lady walking her schnauzer.

The top of Lily's hair bounced in place. She removed the thumb from her kisser, seemed to be speaking. Was something wrong? Just trying to share a thought?

From behind, I couldn't hear a word. Beneath my coat, my shirt was soaked. (I was perpetually soaked with sweat.)

My hip throbbed. I slowed, leaned forward.

Lily repeated her demand. *"Chock-late."*

I answered, "You just had some, love of my life."

"More," she said.

"I thought this was over."

"It's not over. I want *more*."

We passed the college students being paid to solicit pedestrians for charitable contributions.

I ignored them. Aping the lyric of a campy hip-hop smash, I called out: "If there's a problem?"

(During optimal moments, Lily took my prompt, shouting back: "YO, I'll solve it.")

"MORE," she announced.

And here it was, arriving, the dread blumpo.

The real struggle, of course, hits with the fourth time you have to keep control in response to the exact same situation. The eighth time you have to answer that impossible question that was hard enough, forty minutes ago, under the best of circumstances.

The twelfth consecutive time. When you modeled deep breathing. When you followed the advice from parenting websites and changed the subject. When ghosts and grief were crowding your every moment, and you were *still* looking down the barrel of that impossible question, *still* had to try to tailor an answer to your child.

Did I understand that tantrums were a manifestation of fear as much as they were from emotional hurt and physical pain?

Pushing the stroller over an uneven, cracked part of that sidewalk, I deliberately gave some extra *ummph*.

"DADDY."

Pedestrians, hearing her, gawked.

Lily kept at it. Her voice an accordion, she extended her syllables: "*DADD-DDEEY*," contracted: "*DDDY*."

What was my offending issue? My original sin? I'll tell you.

When we'd stopped at the bodega, I'd cut off her Tootsie Roll intake at three.

THAT NIGHT WE magically survived the blumpos, made it to bedtime. She was in her jammies, nestled safely under the covers. Her arm was sticking out, slack atop the comforter, holding her stuffed doll whose full length switched, transforming from the Wicked Witch into Dorothy.

"I'm so sorry about today," I said.

"Whortoo," she answered.

"What was that, sweetie?"

She jumbled syllables, sounding tired. "I want Whortoo and the eleff egg."

I also was beat, in no mood to decipher. "It's late." I stroked her hair. "Maybe just one book."

35

I picked from near the top of the bedside pile, a bright yellow, slim hardback—a book I'd loved as a child. She shook it off. *Curious George Gets Exploited by a White Male Colonialist* landed on the floor.

Lily fought a yawn. Tiny hands reached. One of her go-to moves: she pulled up my shirt to expose my tummy. A giggle. She began tracing along the thick black lines orbiting my belly button: a heart, a sunburst.

We both knew this meant she wanted the magical story of my stomach tattoo. She wanted to hear that her mother had a corresponding image, filled with sunny orange and yellow colors, on the back of her neck.

I thought about it. "I know I promised. That's a long one."

Her hand moved over my arm to a different piece of ink: a lily blossom surrounded by small stars.

"Okay. This one celebrates *your* birth," I said. "See, here is the *Lily*. These are the *stars*. Your name is—"

"Lily Starr."

"Correct-a-mundo, Little Bundo."

All this love put too much nervous energy in her body. Maybe she just needed something to do. Either way, a lazy kick, her foot smacked against the closest wall.

Another one, establishing a little rhythm.

Near the top of that wall, some planks had been nailed and were used as storage shelves. With kick four, kick six, the deluge began— the fall and fall and fall. Gibbon's *History of the Decline and Fall of the Holy Roman Empire*. However many volumes there were, they were doorstops, thick and heavy, every one of them.

In the split second I had to react, I raised my forearm in front of my face, as if trying to block out the rays of the sun.

Pain was a solid mass, filling my reconstructed elbow, my bicep, up to my shoulder, into my ears.

When I could again see in focus, I was screaming. A scream not just from the depths of my lungs, but from somewhere deeper, more primal.

Her eyes were large. Her lip trembling. Her facial features gone fire-truck red.

"Sweetie," I said.

Her mouth opened, that impossible moment before it all comes out.

"*I'm sorry!*" I tried.

Too late. Neck veins jerking. Screaming now, twelve alarms, full blood murder, screaming until her screams stopped producing sound, until she could not breathe. I thought she was going to choke.

I started rubbing her chest, circular motions with my palm, something her mom used to do to calm her.

"It's okay," I said. "It's *okay*."

My voice became calming, though my words still came fast: "I'm sorry. Daddy's sorry. No more losing my temper."

I brought her into me, pressed her into my chest.

"Daddy has to do better," I said. "I know. Daddy will do better."

She made eye contact, sniffled a bit.

"It's not fair."

"Nobody meant anything," I said. "It was just accidents."

"No," Lily said. "Mommy."

Just south of her, a fallen hardback was splayed open; I registered that its typeset print was myopically small, but could read the title of the chapter, larger, referring to the death of an emperor named Severus.

"You're right, it's not fair."

"But why?"

"You have every right to be angry," I said, relying on my forever answer, words my therapist, Dr. Roberts, had provided. "You have every right to be sad."

"*Why?*"

"It is not your fault. It is not anybody's fault."

"Where is Mommy?"

"I don't know. I think Mommy might be up in the sky."

"Can we visit her?"

"The sky is very large."

Lily's voice was soft. "I would search every cloud."

YOU LIE NEXT to your daughter on the bed in the dark and feel the entirety of your obliteration. Seconds pass; somehow, this life does not end. With your head turned off to the side, away from her, she can't see that your eyes are misty. You notice, in a wet blur, that the inks in that rock poster glow in the dark. Their effect may be smeared, but it's still psychedelic: the neon green monster, the radiant pink pixie girl. You stare at the poster and feel breath entering into your body again and you suck in this new oxygen, and gain enough strength, and you turn back onto your other side and look, and keep looking: your daughter's lids fluttering, shutting, the final spasms wracking her body, those last traces of her energy draining, her form going placid, spreading out—as always—all over Mommy's side of the bed.

How long I stared that night at the moony perfection of her profile, I cannot report. How long it took me to put myself back together, I similarly do not know. But eventually I did rise from the bed, onto the balls of my feet, so as not to wake her. In the low light of evening, I scraped away the remains of her uneaten mac and cheese, washed by hand my few dishes and pots. I scarfed down veggie Pirate's Booty, tried without success to get marker stains off the couch. I laid out two cute outfits for her to select from in the morning (thereby helping her develop her own fashion sense). I used a straightened paper clip to withdraw the penny from inside my laptop's DVR mechanism, which, earlier in the day, had been *someone's* version of trying to insert a compact disc. I watched a You-Tube video about how to braid an oversized Barbie skull, but did not practice those steps. I thought for a count about reading a parenting blog, and instead scanned websites for deals on slept-on basketball sneakers. In the reflection of my dozing laptop screen, I examined whether my hairline was receding from the temples. Leaving the apartment and going to the bodega for a soda was categorically out. Going down to the basement to put in laundry was pushing it. Taking the trash down, leaving her alone for three minutes, was that doable? I decided not to risk any of it, spent my energy busting out sets of prison-style stomach crunches, doing weird weight-bearing stretches on my late wife's yoga mat. I sucked air. I focused so my vision would stop being double, then stared at the orange wooden modules, stacked upon one another, that I'd found on the curb a few summers ago, right after NYU's term ended, when students moved home. The wooden modules served as a bookshelf, and on the middle shelf, specifically, I stared at that velvet box, bigger and sturdier than a shoebox, containing the urn with Diana's ashes.

Okay. We weren't under the well. Maybe we weren't even *in* the well anymore.

Even so, there was a pounding. I could hear it: the war drum from the other side of the tree line. Its sound was getting louder, always, closing in.

I don't want this. I don't.

CHAPTER FOUR

"It's about my kids. I want to outlive my children, of course, one hundred percent."

—MMA legend Tito Ortiz

FORTY-FIVE MINUTES BEFORE Lily's big debut. I was idling in the lobby of the dance center, resplendent in a rumpled shirt and sample sale jeans that kind of fit, holding the bouquet of overpriced lilies that I'd purchased from a bodega down the street. The lobby, empty when I'd arrived, was now adult-contemporary rocking, with wives and hubbies crowding around the inner entrance, angling to get in when the doors opened, grab the best seats. Scattered around were a few of the women I'd sat with, in this place's basement, on Wednesday afternoons, all of us observing our beginners through one-way glass, with me particularly focused on the far end of the ballet bar, Lily tugging at her leotard, Lily checking in the full-length wall of mirrors to see how she looked.

My phone's pictures from that afternoon show an out-of-focus, bluish-purple blur on a stage among other little blurs, her arms stretched to full length above her head. Turns out, Lily stood on her tippy toes, twirled, and danced for all of six minutes—off-the-chart adorable minutes, yes, but six of them. More pictures show her beaming afterward, laughing, hugging a bunch of other girls who we'd never see again, all of them joyous. My child remained energized that day, full to the brim with wiggles.

Cut to Madison Square Park. Four in the afternoon. This was a weekend, meaning despite that spring's weird chilly stretch, the playground was packed to the figurative rafters, with eight-year-olds causing all kinds of hell on the toddler slides. Some Euro tourist had made the mistake of bringing a special toy with their sweet darling, and a bunch of the other toddlers were crying, wanting to claim that prize. My child—coat unzipped, purple leotard revealed in flashes—chased after a trio of girls who most definitely did not want to play with her.

Off to the side, I stood by some fence, away from all the other parents, trying to stay afloat, hoping to survive until dinner. My eyes wandered, checking the sidelines for any young moms. A requisite cluster of upscale professional women were ignoring their little dearies, gabbing with other upscale professional women, comparing the sugar content of various organic yogurt pouches. Fathers ideal enough to be ordered from a catalogue were showing all kinds of pep, bouncing around the jungle gym (easy enough; they only had to spend stretches of thirty concentrated minutes with Champ during weekends). One family unit was reassembling nearby, their jocular pal unstacking cardboard boxes of Shake Shack for everyone. Weather-resistant squirrels were stalking unsuspecting innocents for cheese fries. The sky was a collection of fat clouds the color of concrete. Children kept running, climbing, swinging, heading down slides, their laughter audible from every direction.

The great majority of my life had been spent feeling alone, but the aloneness I felt in these moments was so deep, I was forced to stand face-to-face with it.

MY MOTHER, CARYL Ida Starr, is the daughter of second-generation immigrants. (Her grandparents came over from Austria.) She graduated from the Bronx High School of Science, a special public school for high achieving students, when she was sixteen. In modern times, she would have been on the fast track to an Ivy; in the 1950s, though, even the smartest women usually ended up as switchboard operators, teachers, nurses. My mother was no exception: she attended Queens College, where she earned both a degree and a teaching certificate. At a dance on the Lower East Side, she met Howard Bock, a tall brown-eyed boy from the Lower East Side who told her he'd tried out for the New York Yankees. The couple fell for each other, married, and soon moved to Las Vegas, partially in the hopes the dry weather would help Mother's mom fight her lung cancer, partially so my dad could find regular employment. (The Yankees had never called back.) With a growing family to look after, my mother needed flexible hours, so she worked as a substitute teacher and Tupperware saleswoman; my father dealt craps on the strip.

I was the third of four. Among the things I remember from my childhood are the sound of planes from the airport passing above our home, swirling wallpaper patterns in our kitchen, transparent plastic over the couch, my mom cooking us tongue for dinner—like, once a week or so—and that before I knew better, I actually liked the bumpy sensation of the meat's underside in my mouth. The merciless summer sun beat down on me and my two older brothers while we rummaged around vacant lots, fruitlessly hunting for lizards amid the tumbleweeds and sand. When my brothers left me and played ball with their friends, which happened a good deal of the time, Crystal and I engaged in backyard fantasies with forts and trees, or put on living room shows together (usually for our dolls and toys). Each July Fourth the entire family drove around in our station wagon and looked up through the windshield and watched for blooming fireworks in the endless Nevada sky. On nights of big championship fights, my dad chauffeured me, my brothers, and my sister up and down the freeway next to the strip. Every three minutes, local radio reports cut in with action from the most recent round. Whenever we passed Caesars Palace, all of us pushed to the nearest window and gawked at the makeshift stadium that had been built in the parking lot and listened to the crowd's roar, trying to spot the fighters.

Those are a few early childhood memories. They are uniformly warm.

I was around seven years old when my dad borrowed money to take over a struggling pawnshop downtown, off Fremont Street, a move that changed the direction of our lives. Downtown Vegas in the eighties was a lot like Times Square during its famed porno phase, a gritty, even scummy area. Working in a downtown Vegas pawnshop might have been a lively and unique profession, but it also was a grind, and more than a little soul numbing. My mother and father toiled alongside each other in that pawnshop, seven days a week, ten hours a day, closing the store only for Yom Kippur.

This ended our financial woes. We moved out of that small home by the airport, to a suburban split-level, but this was Vegas, and, as with any Vegas transaction, there had to be a price. No small part of a pawnbroker's job is helping people who are down of their luck. My dad was an amiable expert on that front, happy to make small talk, to try and negotiate a deal. At the same time, discerning what a person *really* wanted is a paramount aspect of the pawnbroker's job. By necessity, my parents learned to view every work conversation through a cynical lens: *How is this mamzer trying to rip me off?*

Pawnshop Lady. The single last job on earth suited to the particularly tenderhearted, brilliant, nervous woman who is my mother.

Her eyes—puppy brown, vulnerable, oceanic in their depth—didn't just seek you out; they also sucked you in. (I'm pretty sure Lily got her large, wide eyes from my mother.) More than a few friends have marveled over my mother's powerful gaze; making eye contact, they'd felt a sudden intense connection with her. And it's true: there was this big needy part of her, looking for connection, wanting to take you into her confidence. The problem was that, as a rule, she remained suspicious before anything, a woman deeply distrustful of people, places, the whole wide world.

A few events had exacerbated this fissure, the main one being that my mom had four kids in a span of three years. (My brothers are older than me by two years and twins; my sister is a year younger than me.) Raising four kids on limited funds in the wild and unrelenting West will drive anybody up a tree. Let's just assume this to be true. Throw in that my third-grade teacher learned about the pawnshop from a stray remark I made and soon after started pawning jewelry with my folks. On top of that, not a year later, a boy who'd attended the same Hebrew school as me and my siblings—he was a bit behind us; we did not know him—was abducted from the school grounds and never found. (It was national news; his abductors to this day remain at large.) Again, worth restating: this was Vegas in the late seventies. My mother looked at the cards on the table and made the natural play—at least, the play natural to her. She ordered: No longer could we tell teachers, friends, or anyone, what our parents did. She wasn't going to take a chance on us being abducted. For the rest of my childhood, our parents were in *sales*.

Crystal and I had bedrooms next to one another, but we had different paths. When she was twelve or so, she started dying her hair blue, smoking clove cigarettes out of her window and smashing the butts in the sill, so she wouldn't get caught; she used to sneak out of the house, meet up with older friends. By contrast, fourteen-year-old me was isolated in my room, reading comic books, wishing I was the one with superpowers. Nonetheless, like victims who'd survived the same traumatic events, Crystal and I bonded over the way Mother used to barge into our respective rooms; we called her the hurricane. Five, six in the morning, the hurricane's brain would have been in overdrive all night and she'd need to unburden herself. This could mean reminding me (or Crystal) how to handle the tricky point of that day's test. It could mean arguing some imaginary slight she'd heard from the waiter during the previous night's dinner (after work at a casino coffee shop). It could mean relitigating some point of a dispute that the rest of the world had long forgotten. Something I'd done, something my brothers had done.

Our mother also was convinced people whispered conspiracies about her. Anyone being overly polite got her nervous. An undefeated champion at rejecting before being rejected, she felt white-tablecloth restaurants were too fancy for her, and refused to step inside them. For no good reason, she erupted at cashiers, at shoe salesmen. "They should do me a favor and drop dead" was a phrase she often mumbled to herself, after the fact, while driving us home. Like so many immigrants and children of immigrants, so many people who found themselves outsiders, she also possessed a searing need for approval, asking, during the course of my life, some version of *What did your teacher think? Did your professor like it? What does your editor say?*

And then there was her true go-to, used when she was deeply upset and could not get us kids to calm down: "*I wish I had never been born.*"

I've talked with my siblings about this last one. Each of us heard it a little differently, Crystal in particular. Understand, during her high school years, my sister's rebellion had evolved, channeled through all-night prep sessions, manifesting in statewide awards in rhetoric and drama. Upon turning eighteen, she'd turned down scholarships out west to study acting in Manhattan (also heading east, probably, to get out from under Mom's shadow). Relentlessly positive, forever pushing back against Vegas's baked-in cynicism, converting that hardness into an almost breathtaking ability to sympathize, Crystal resolutely believes that our mother's remark—"*I wish I'd never been born*"—is an expression of a woman overwhelmed, a woman not wanting to be in the fix of raising four kids and working the hours she did, not wanting this life of sale rack clothing and secondhand stereos and haggling with inveterate gamblers.

I am sure my sister is correct. But my ears—less secure, more prone to brooding—heard a different sentence: *I wish you had never been born*. I heard my mother wishing she had not had me.

Here's one more line, used when our mother felt we weren't taking school seriously, when we were disappointing her: "Don't you see? We're doing this so you won't have to."

Show me a person who does everything out of duty, I'll show you one furious human.

MEET NINA! THE latest in our revolving door of sitters and erstwhile nannies! Originally from Portugal and ostensibly in the United States to study performance art! Showing herself to be a performance in her own right! Hair a succulent orange bob! Grotesquely oversized eyewear that, remarkably, still accentuated her sharp features! Flannel shirt enveloping her like a yurt! Denim overalls, cuffs rolled with a precision that appeared military! Calf-high Docs! She justified the exclamation marks: her total effect that of a young woman working diligently and successfully to be striking. At once wholly efficient and impossibly funky.

Bending into a crouch, Nina made eye contact with Lily, placed a manicured hand onto Lily's shoulder. "Do you enjoy music?"

Lily, awestruck, nodded.

"I do too. Do you want to be my friend?"

Lily didn't respond.

"Let me tell you this: *If you don't like Blonde Redhead, you cannot be my friend.*"

Lily thought. "I like Blonde Redhead."

Nina's smile was generous and, at the same time, plotting mayhem; she revealed excellent canines.

"Daddy!" Lily turned toward me. "If you don't like Blondehead, Daddy, you cannot be my friend!"

Thus, the reins of the stroller were handed over, Nina joining the crew, coming on full-time as Lily's babysitter. A normal family had parents tagging in, providing needed breaks, taking turns being the bad cop, delivering the necessary heart-to-heart, each parent acting both as confidant to the child and as ballast for and against one another; in this home, Nina strategized about how to get Lily to stop sucking her thumb. Nina goaded and teased Lily into eating her broccoli; she instructed Lily through projects that involved significant quantities of water and flour, modeled the latest cool dances, then captured, on her phone, Lily's flailing imitations. Nina tapped into reservoirs of positive energy previously untapped in my child. I saw how Lily looked forward to her showing up each morning, and I also watched how, returning from one day trip to Central Park and a museum, Nina spoke to Lily in clipped, one- and two-word sentences, making sure Lily took off her shoes, washed her hands. Afterward, Nina let me know how much money she'd spent on their lunch and that she'd wait while I went to the bank machine. Nina made sure to inform me when she had an exam and would have to leave here early.

Then came the day I could see that Nina's shoulders were slumped, her gas tank empty.

They'd returned from the playground on Second Avenue. Something was on her mind.

She mentioned a little steel counter in the playground. I knew it well. Amid the mandated slides and bridges, it sort of looked like an open-air window space, with metal bars running up each side. Lily enjoyed putting her head in the space, playing storekeeper.

"Is cute, you know?" Nina said. "I ask to buy strawberry ice cream. Lily answers, 'We are out.' I say, 'Vanilla.' 'We are out.' Every flavor are out."

"Right," I said, saving a document on my laptop.

"The market is out of everything." Nina undid the final button of her glittery thrift store cardigan. "I pretend the counter is for clock store. Lily says clocks are broken. I tell Lily I want to buy two broken clocks. No. 'We're out of the broken clocks.'"

"The anecdote's definitely charming, Nina."

"I am bringing this up for a reason, Charles."

I turned toward her.

"I am Lily's advocate. She does something, you get upset, I don't think is a big deal, I tell you. *This is acting normal.*"

"Right," I said. Now she had my attention.

"Refusing to eat the peanut butter and jelly," Nina said. "I seen this before. Sometimes it is flirt. Sometimes confrontation. But is what the little ones must do in order to express. Part of the growing process. Remember, I was nanny for two years in Lisbon."

"Something's up?" I said.

Nina worked her nose into a kind of scowl. She thought about what to say next, but instead rubbed at the back of her hamstring, as if this could ease her growing frustration. "I don't know yet."

ON THE FIRST Saturday afternoon of June, in the hopes of expressing our appreciation for Nina—her calming presence, the normalcy she'd imported to our home—Lily and I purchased a cheap bottle of wine, then headed down into the full diaper known as the Manhattan subway system. All the lines we needed were out of service or under construction, but we would not be deterred, soldiering on, sweating, waiting for new and obscure transfers, discovering new and exciting body odors.

Dehydrated, sweating, cranky, we emerged onto the mean streets of deepest, newly gentrified Bushwick, and made our way to the open studios, the studio walk, whatever you want to call what was taking place in a converted factory whose elevators were not in service. Fifth floor; requisite corrugated metal pipes and brick and concrete; mandatorily dim studio; casting call–provided hipsters—fifteen or twenty, figure, most of them seated on the cement. Across the room was a makeshift stage. A performance was underway: someone in a goatee producing tortured sounds on a theremin, flailing interpretive dancers, some de rigueur spoken-word bullshit.

My daughter immediately recognized the young woman in the middle of the stage. Lily broke free from my grip and rushed.

"NINA. NINA."

Lily climbed onto the stage. Lily resisted attempts to get her down—first from *"NINA,"* then other cast members. She refused to budge, adding to the afternoon's performance with her own, one that turned howling, if not satanic.

Picture, if you will, the aftermath of this ruined masterpiece, as captured in a children's picture book. Believe me, if I had talent, I'd draw it for you: musical stands and a chair knocked over, the theremin player/hipsters at the cheese table commiserating, maybe some wires and speakers in the back. Meanwhile, a happily oblivious Lily (adorned in a small pair of overalls) holds Nina's hand, eats a cookie.

Nina, wearing a ridiculous performance outfit (maybe a leotard?), speaks to/lectures an apologetic Charles (hoodie). Nina has a serious expression. Her free hand is in a fist, positioned on her shapely hip. Her dialogue bubble says:

"Have you ever thought of having Lily talk to someone?"

BEING TOLD THAT your three-year-old daughter might be in the throes of mental distress is no-shit horrific.

My first instinct was to deny, avoid, close my ears.

But there was no avoiding the experience of Lily's defiance, no way to deny the vortex of her tantrums.

All too well, I knew that my mother should have spent her adulthood on meds. Her life would have been better. My dad's life would have been easier. All of our lives would have benefited.

My dad's older brother, when he'd been in class at graduate school at Columbia, had suffered a psychotic break. It had affected his ability to think and care for himself, and for the rest of his life, his parents had to support him; when they were too old, my dad took over the bills, while his sister coordinated the logistics of his care. Meaning there were issues on my father's side too.

I'd been something of the remaindered middle child: my older brothers were athletes with outsized personalities and problems, while my sister was the family's darling and star. Which is to say, I didn't quite get the attention I wanted from my parents. I was also a late bloomer, one of those kids who's always a step behind in junior high school, trying to figure out just who those bands on the concert T-shirts that other kids wore were, why I couldn't I ever find that music on the radio. At best I was the third-smallest boy in my public high school. What in God's name was I doing trying out for the high school basketball team? I had faith; my ballhandling skills would impress; similarly, the sharp and worthwhile kids would learn I was bighearted and interesting, possessing good taste in television shows and a honed sense of humor that extended into irony, absurdity, even dry wit. But let's be real. My malnourished ass was never going to wrangle a spot at the end of the varsity bench, and the scions of dealers and cowboys and Mormons and young Jewish Vegas mafiosi, sure as molasses is slow, they weren't going to value, let alone embrace, any sort of witticism from of my pimpled mug. And so, instead of wearing a letterman's jacket, having a girlfriend, going on a date, or even stealing a single kiss during my high school years; instead of being invited to parties and keggers and rooms with a circle of kids passing around doobage—instead of showing off my true and radiant self—I spent a whole lot of time walking the dog at night with my mom.

In modern times, it would be easy for this version of me to burrow my way toward 4Chan and other back channels. And in eighties Vegas, it's regrettably true to report, I followed that template to some degree, sort of existing on the periphery. I was a know-it-all, distrustful of society and authority. I had problems following orders, and was far more likely to make a dismissive remark than embrace the unfamiliar. But I never fully descended into conspiracy theories and incel culture. Maybe I wasn't a fully demonstrative bleeding heart like my sister; nonetheless, my humanist defense systems, meager though they might have been, remained on alert, responding to the empathetic parts of what went on in pawnshops, moving me away from the nasty confrontations my parents got into with customers. That humane instinct—the one that pleaded for my parents to always act first with decency—remained curious, interested in the well-being of others. I may not have fully understood how someone assimilates into the culture at large. I definitely did not want to submit and *fit in.* But something inside urged me to push back against my chaotic feelings, to find ways to quell them.

This search continued as an undergrad. While I was working on the school newspaper, in the middle of one editorial meeting, our staff advisor—a wonderful journalist named Gary Libman—noticed everyone lagging. Instead of being confrontational, he waited. The next week, when the meeting reached its midpoint, he asked all of us to stand up, stretch, shake out our arms, get some water if we needed it. This made a massive impression on me. Instead of blindly barging straight ahead, instead of indulging my desire for attention, or concentrating only on what I wanted, instead of taking stray remarks as insults, instead of overreacting, lashing out, and just Bocking things up, perhaps I could learn how to recognize the larger reality of what was happening in front of me and respond accordingly, to listen to what someone was *actually* saying.

I felt certain there was a better life for me, that I could *evolve* my way toward accomplishment, toward acceptance. With that in mind, whatever meager ambitions I possessed evolved in a specific way. That same exasperated mantra my mother shouted to push me, without success, toward better grades—"We're doing this so you won't have to"—transmogrified, becoming further justification, first for not settling for an office job, then for not buying into the ownership society. Instead, I granted myself permission to follow weird dreams, scrounging along on the fringes—as a low-rung sportswriter in Mississippi, a graduate student going back and forth from New York to Vermont, an aspiring novelist—relying on my self-proclaimed truths long past the point where validation was coming my way, where there were tangible reasons to suggest my supposed talents would make good. Similarly, my mother's wish (whether or not she'd actually wished I'd never been born, that's what I heard, omnipresent, crystalline) had me perpetually chasing gold stars. Even as I felt myself coming up short, I kept trying to prove I was worthy of an invitation to the proverbial kegger, a date for the prom, a mother's love.

"He wants awfully to be inside staring out: anybody with their nose pressed against a glass is liable to look stupid," says Holly Golightly about the narrator in Truman Capote's *Breakfast at Tiffany's*. Reader, I routinely looked worse than stupid. Diana, Crystal, and more than a few others had let me know through the years: I possessed no clue how harsh my reactions could get, nor of the sheer range of my repertoire for expressing derision—squinting and jutting my jaw; staring death at someone who did not do what I wanted the moment I wanted it; turning my face to stone in such a way that it let the person who'd just spoken know that it was a miracle they'd figured out how to say words in the first place; twisting my expression into a rictus of hateful red-hot liquid nuclear obliteration; or just turning inward, but inward in a way so that all life was extinguished, all ambition, all hope, all feeling, and the only thing left was the emanated desire to be doing anything other than dealing with this *bullshit*.

Nobody consciously wants to be that guy.

And nobody wants the possibility that their little girl might be on her way, might be echoing these awful traits.

THE FIVE BOROUGHS of New York City represent a universe that works on its own terms. Among these terms is the one where Manhattan child therapists don't accept health insurance. Calls revealed theirs was a cash-centric biz, with rates starting at three hundred an hour. A dive into the web uncovered a support group for youths who'd lost a mom to cancer; the catch, you had to be at least five years old to join. (Let's acknowledge, up there among the roughest collection of syllables: *an age requirement for the grieving youth cancer support group.*)

Opening his address book, my therapist, Mark Roberts, dictated to me the phone number of a center: the William Alanson White Institute. They trained counselors to specialize in children's therapy. "The center's graduates are building their patient lists. Sometimes they offer special rates."

This is how, toward the end of June, I was able to get Lily started: Jennifer Melfi, let's call her. A kind woman, early thirties, maybe, always giving off a proper, respectable vibe—matching jacket and skirt, a loose blouse and jeans. She shared an office in the West Twenties with other therapists.

The Saturday afternoon we arrived, Lily wore stylish pink shades, a matched plaid dress, and sparkly pink shoes. Dr. Melfi complimented her on her outfit. Lily brushed back her hair. "Thank you. I picked it out myself."

I stayed in the office while they got comfortable. Lily began to look at the different toys, took out a jar of Play-Doh. She brought it closer to Dr. Melfi, sat on the floor with her.

Lily and Dr. Melfi played dolls, I would learn, eventually.

Lily sometimes had her dolls take the Play-Doh and build ladders to reach the sky, I would also learn.

One Saturday a few weeks later, from her stroller, as we headed home from a session, Lily told me that Jennifer needed to buy more Play-Doh. There wasn't enough to get to all the clouds.

They also played with the dollhouse in Dr. Melfi's office. Lily had the doctor take on the mom character. Lily then instructed the mom to yell at the girl doll for being bad. For not listening. The girl was ordered to sleep in the garage, to clean the roof all day.

Lily showed herself to Dr. Melfi as strong-willed, bright, fiery, loving. She showed herself to be normal in many ways, but also as wrestling with denial about Diana's death, wrestling with guilt, and blaming herself. The girl doll was bad even as the mom doll was pretty, perfect, endlessly kind. Dr. Melfi sometimes took the girl doll's side during the play sessions, and protested: sleeping in the garage seemed a harsh punishment for not listening. It wasn't easy to listen all the time.

Lily's response was to have a dog figure join the girl in the doghouse. The girl and the dog got to be together. Then Lily added, for Dr. Melfi, "Make sure you lock up this house so no other kids can come."

There wasn't enough insight yet for definitive answers. Lily's psyche was still forming and it was hard to get specific about the severity of her feelings. But this much was plain: when we got to the bus stop just as the bus started pulling away; when I couldn't read on the throne for five minutes without *someone* tapping on the door and calling, repeatedly, for me; when I'd finally put on and secured her sneakers and she let out a pained cry and I saw they were on the wrong feet; when I entered that space where I looked at her and the only thing I could think to do was wipe her mouth, take whatever thing out of her grip, ask her to put that away; when I hadn't bathed her for a few days and then sprayed her hair with de-tangler and she grabbed the brush right out of my hands and insisted she could do her own hair; when we reached a massive knot that I could not get the comb through and her screams outpaced anything I'd anticipated; when I muttered, "*Mother fuck*"; when she kept bawling; when I felt she was sort of milking it and I stopped with the comb and stared out at the ether and could not help myself and said, "*Oh, just fuck me*"; when I saw her eyes twitch, saw this little wisp of a child slumping, buckling, and once again, too late, realized that *I* was the instigator? That shit had to stop. I had to do better.

I look back on all this—again, from a safe distance of ten years later—and I see that I was too inside our daily grind to have any perspective, specifically with regards to my grief and how it might have been affecting our daily lives. I sure wasn't thinking big picture, for instance, about the lineage of mental instability on both sides of my family history, how *that* might have been affecting my ability to handle fatherhood and widowhood. Nor was I considering the cornucopia of lingering and unresolved issues from my early years, let alone how they might have resulted in a damaged inner child who was, himself, nowhere near ready to care for an actual real-world little girl.

I similarly was not thinking about how formative and destructive my negative influence could be for Lily. I was not thinking about Lily's unspoken grief, how it might have been rotting her from the inside. Not about the toxic combination of this laundry list of factors or how potent this toxicity might have been.

What I do remember thinking incessantly, in loops, returning to, using as a mantra, is that what I could do—what I was doing—was to keep on my grind. The apartment was rent-stabilized, so I didn't have a huge overhead. We had health insurance for a while thanks to the Authors Guild, a little money still left from the advance for the new book, and my publishing house would cough up more, should two hundred new pages magically appear. I'd also become mobile enough to teach an undergraduate writing workshop in the fall, so that would mean a few more pennies. I had Mondays to Fridays, when Lily was with Nina, to teach and write and try and figure out how to pay the bills. Lily had Saturdays from 3:00 to 3:50 p.m. with Dr. Melfi to get deep. Sunday mornings the two of us trekked across town to the West Village: I kvetched to Crystal about my latest misadventures in fatherhood. She answered right back about being a mom to a young child and whether she'd ever be able to get auditions again. We snacked and supervised, laughed and unwound; Lily and her cousin, Declain, scarfed organic juice boxes from my sister's fridge, chased each other around the block, and dug around in the local playground's sandbox. In my mind's eye, I still see Crystal pleasantly calling out something to Lily, my child listening, following instructions, looking to her aunt for more guidance.

On Sunday evenings, after we returned home and rested a bit, Susannah took over, coming by to get Lily and venture back out into the city, the two going out for dinner, maybe shopping for something fun, then returning, for now it was time for their special Skype sessions with Grandma Peg. Here were Peg's snow-white hair and kind eyes coming into focus on my laptop.

Admittedly, proper etiquette would have been to chat with my dead wife's mom, spend three whole minutes trading niceties. By that time of night, though, I was spent. I mumbled something toward the laptop, then stumbled into the bedroom. After all, tomorrow there were dance classes to get her to, gymnastics across town. Depending on how the calendar played out, there were friends stopping by, day trips needing coordination, museum visits, lollipop runs, Nina filling me in, rescheduled appointments, impromptu pop-ins from out of the fucking sky, all of us giving it every bit of what we were supposed to, trying to feed a child's wonder and delight, filling in new areas of the jigsaw puzzle that was her sense of this world, in short, manifesting the idea of a mother's love through our piece-by-piece effort, our growing infrastructure, and, okay, it wasn't a replacement, not close, but still . . .

CHAPTER FIVE

THAT FALL, WE had what, on first, second, and fourth glance, appeared to be an upgrade to our circumstances.

Those letters of recommendation that Crystal had harassed me into chasing down, way back when I'd been on the couch, recovering from my accident? Those letters ended up unlocking doors to the administrative offices of no fewer than three pre-kindergarten and day care centers. And once these doors were unlocked, Lily must have done pretty well at her subsequent playdate interview things (in which said administrators watched her and other kids interacting). Probably the ins and outs of our super-sad sob story helped here and there. However it happened, the end result was Lily being enrolled in the preschool arm of the Third Street Music School Settlement.

Third Street Music School Settlement: the longest running community music school in the United States—servicing young and adult musicians alike since 1890-whenever. Actually located on East Eleventh Street and not its original Third Street location, meaning closer to us and easier to wheel Lily to and from (huzzah!). Four stories of red brick that looked transported straight from the nineteenth century, only with the building updated, the bricks scrubbed and welcoming, more like a gentrified Dickens and not a scary orphanage (another huzzah!). They also housed an elementary school, as well as kindergarten and toddler programs—which, let's be honest, helped keep the lights on. We qualified for their toddler financial aid package, almost making Lily's school year affordable.

It felt monumental, getting her to this moment, this place, providing her the chance to enter into a routine, to have an organized, socializing structure. I felt like I should be performing a live ritual sacrifice to show my thankfulness—although, now that I think of it, Lily in pre-K meant sacrificing Nina. There wouldn't be enough hours to make employing her worthwhile. This was definitely a loss: Nina's presence had added feminine joy and stability to Lily's life. But it was also apparent, Nina had been exhausted by her summer; she was ready for something new.

From the department of self-interest, I was too. Most of the writers who'd published books around the time of my first novel had already published new books. They were winning awards, getting tenure, and selling television shows. In down moments, occasionally, I responded like any reasonable person and searched the magic Google machine for updates of my peers' successes. I knew I wasn't going to be on a career fast track anytime soon—most likely that dream was gone—but with Lily in school, at least I'd be able to designate set hours when I got to visit my writing space in Union Square, a third-floor communal area divvied into cubicles. (Figure, ink-stained wretches toiling on manuscripts and screenplays, also arguing—politely, fervently—about the best percentages for dark chocolate.) I'd be able to spread out at a desk, occupy my own head for a bit. I could commit to the process of writing, recovering this part of myself.

"What if I don't make friends," she asked. "What if the teacher doesn't like me?"

I answered her concerns by showing her a picture book: the story of a longtime teacher who was nervous on the night before school started. I asked if she understood.

She cuddled into me, stayed there a long time.

"Another bedtime story," she said.

"Which one, sweetheart?"

"Elefegg."

"I keep telling you, I don't know that one."

"Hotor."

"I'll keep checking for Hotor."

She studied me. *I am so disappointed in you, Daddy, but keep trying to understand.*

We sang our eighties medley. We stared up into the dark at our Day-Glo cosmos. We visualized waves, first crashing on the beach, then heading back out into the ocean. The next morning I slipped out of the new pack that I'd purchased, and onto her narrow body, a clean, new white pair of underpants with a small pink flower on the front. I helped her ease into the sleeves of a purple frock that I'd liberated from the dreck of a Daffy's sale rack. We got on her glittery gray tights, Ugg-ish pink boots. Combing her hair, lightly, so it did not hurt too bad, I twisted her scrunchie so she had a neat ponytail.

Saved from my phone, pictures show Lily strapped into her stroller, staring up at me and the camera phone. Her eyes are doubtful, her mouth twisted in an expression that might be sarcastic, maybe a bit shy.

No school wants the little ones overwhelmed during that inaugural week. Which meant Lily's first day at Third Street lasted all of one hour. To a child, though, it's still the first day, still the unknown. At the cusp of the classroom, Lily waited, going quiet. Other kids were already in the classroom, gathered at different tables, grabbing things, talking. She'd only had that week of camp at the Y; was this too much for her? She took her time, walked into the room, soon enough sought out a table of art supplies. She did not look up at me, kept playing with the green clay, did not notice when I called her name or waved goodbye.

INSTEAD OF HEADING to the writing space—I had only an hour, what was the point?—I grabbed a bagel, returned to the school ten or so minutes early. The small courtyard in front was laid out with rubber carpeting, allowing the area to serve as a playground. Just inside the fenced perimeter, a new curveball caught me looking, buckled my knees.

Mommies. Maybe two dozen. Wearing light fall coats, fashionably large sweaters. Well-meaning. Caring. Occupying the wooden benches and standing around. Supremely competent in so many walks of life. Most were first-time parents and therefore on edge about their kids—their energy radiated, palpable, potentially ravenous, yet at the same time was being held back, for the moment translating into lots of plastic smiles, tight nodding.

These days, thanks to prestige TV shows like HBO's *Big Little Lies*, the daily procession—all those mothers waiting at the schoolyard—has become a recognized cultural happening. I had no clue about it, but, suspicious, kept away from their gaggles, clutched the wilted cheese stick in my pocket.

The building doors opened outward. Leading the way were the teaching pair, each in her late fifties, one with dark curly hair, the other flowing white. Toddlers followed—a dozen, two dozen— toddling, stumbling, too cute for words, down the middle of a cement path in a polite, orderly, almost straight line. It seemed to me that each emerging child raised his or her head, seeking out Mommy. Then sprinted, hugged.

Of course, Lily was near the back.

When her eyes found me, her relief was transformative: "DADDY!"

Squishy cheese liquefied inside my grip. The tightness in my stomach turned golden. I opened my arms; Lily rushed to me, her words tumbling out—forward rolls, awkward attempted cartwheels, no phrase coming quickly enough: "I get a cubby, we sit at a table, there are four of us—"

She let me hug her, needed to tell me everything, also needed to break away, run around, play in the courtyard, be with her new friends.

HALCYON WEEKS UNFOLDED as if straight from a widower daddy's wish list: Lily followed every instruction given by either of her two teachers; she showed herself as eager to please, kind to other children, enthusiastic about fitting in. At pickup time, my daughter took part in games, breaking off with girls to run, laugh, and chatter with other groups. She made friends, socialized, opening up.

Sitting on one of the benches of the courtyard perimeter, just enough distance from everyone to differentiate myself, mark myself as *separate*, I watched her from my natural, defensive hunch, unable to help myself, half anticipating things going wrong, rooting for her as if I'd bet my life savings on the results. The perimeter of that courtyard was scattered with sitters, there for pickup, some nannies as well. Now and then other dads showed up—invariably scruffy but well-kept, soft in their manners and on their best behavior, working to fit in with the otherwise maternal vibe. Really, though, that playground was a feminine space; specifically, it was a maternal space. Its great majority of occupants were indeed mothers, younger than me, usually. Upscale-ish, new transplants to the East Village, possessors of powerful jobs and faded ankle tattoos and other things to do with their time, but who were in this courtyard with their kiddies, talking shop with other moms, discussing Don Draper's latest Sunday evening transgression.

I silently took in their fall jackets—designer fare manufactured to look more tattered than my legitimately beaten coat. I tossed a nod, gave smiles that I hoped were better than perfunctory.

While Lily was catching her breath, while she circled back on her jaunts, you just know she saw those mommies, too. You best believe she studied their mannerisms. As if pulled along by interior, magnetic forces, Lily gravitated toward their Tupperware containers of prepped pasta and fresh fruit, the care they displayed while delivering forkfuls into their kids' waiting yaps.

LILY HAD BEEN, what, two months old when CUNY started its winter semester; Diana had been raring to go, refusing to take off the semester either for her own final classes or the teaching job that was part of her scholarship package. She was scheduled to instruct Intro to Comp, meaning incoming freshmen whose literacy marks had not measured up—mostly immigrants, first-in-their-families college students who, if they were to stay enrolled, needed the rudimentary elements of what goes into a sentence, a paragraph, an essay. With our baby strapped to her chest, Diana sat on our couch, up through the deepest parts of the night, alternating between feeding and jiggling the child and prepping and fine-tuning her lesson plans. Now and then she'd expound about the importance of doing well by her students, ideas for the opening lecture. I shit you not when I tell you she brought Lily with her, to her classes. I'd volunteered to take care of the little dumpling, but Diana saw that mine was an obligatory offering; she had good reason to doubt my ability to care for an infant, by myself, for an entire afternoon. More important, she did not want be away from Lily, refused to be away from her, instead loading a backpack full of diapers and bottles full of breast milk, taking the stroller with her. Diana hired an undergrad to push the stroller with baby Lily up and down the hallway outside class. At each hour mark during the three-hour class, she'd duck outside to check on them. As soon as the class was done, she came out, grabbed her baby, and resumed her mothering duties.

This was what it meant to be all in. It was what Lily saw from the mothers in that courtyard on a daily basis, what I watched Lily taking in: women with open arms, quick to call out, ready to embrace, eager with pasta, with the right organic juice box, anything that a child could possibly desire, could need, before the child even knew what that might be. I was not one for conscious grief. To be frank, it was hard to make time when there was this toddler to care for, when there was so much to figure out (how we were going to pay bills, deal with three percent of what goes into your average New York minute, yadda yadda yadda). There was a hole inside of me—I knew that much—but I just kept doing my Beckett imitation, shoving my head down, plowing onward, knowing that, fine, my core had this hole, this void. In the courtyard, sitting on the bench, registering Lily registering these mothers, I fell down that void. Just how much Diana would have wanted to be there. How much she would have loved being part of that courtyard, this klatch of mommy conversations. You see those women transcend themselves, elevating into these amazing, powerhouse mothers. I wished I would have gotten to see the powerhouse mom my wife would have become. Of all the people who'd wanted—no, who'd *deserved*—the experience, she had been at the top of the list. This loss, this absence, it overwhelmed me, hurling me further down the void. Who Lily would have grown into under Diana's tutelage? It's something I still wonder about. How the two of them would have been together. What people each of them would have become. All of it, ghost upon ghost. Diana would have done much better than I was doing.

Meanwhile the kids kept on with their cutesy mayhem; the otherwise mundane afternoon continued.

A few moms were grouping nearby. I could not help myself and eavesdropped.

Little Astrid had six stitches right along her right eyebrow from where she'd tumbled down the stairwell. Guthrie smacked his chin against a table edge. Mother after mother documented her kid's scar.

"I feel responsible," one admitted. "I shouldn't, I just do."

"Right," another said. "It's a normal part of being a parent."

Still another: "But it's so hard to give yourself a break. I can't do it."

I kept listening. Maybe scooted a bit toward them.

WOULDN'T IT BE a pleasure to report that the moms sensed my interest, took me into their klatch, walked me to a special backroom coffee shop where you needed a password to get all the billion-dollar mothering secrets? How awesome it would be to let you know, here, that the other kids not just accepted but anointed Lily, fighting over her, who among them was worthy of her deigning to attend their playdate, let alone their sleepover.

Yeah, let's segue.

Third Street's adult conservatory kicked into action and started performing weekly lunchtime concerts for the kiddies. Official-looking adults in black formal wear; mellifluous melodic performances. The combination had its desired effect, and overpowered Lily. Just as impressive to her: the sight of teenagers ambling the school hallways with their stickered cases. The violin didn't simply present itself as a gorgeous instrument to Lily; it became an object of unending interest, one that looked supercool when all the people were jamming on it with those sticks. Possessing the wondrous confidence that comes with being a toddler, Lily had no doubt, she'd be awesome at violin. "I'm almost four. I'm a big girl," she said. "I will practice. I promise."

Today she was trying to keep that promise. The living room window was acting as her backdrop: stuffed bears and unicorns along its ledge, weak, fluttering snowfall on the other side of the pane. Lily was concentrating, fully occupied with her beginner's violin, trying to balance it under her chin. Winter sky toward evening; afternoon's remaining light along the perfect curvature of her cheek. I watched her strain to keep the instrument's body steady. The lit outline of her profile; the structure of Lily's skull appeared to me frail, perfect as an egg. Her head was lowered in such a way that her inherited Bock forehead all but leaped out. For long moments I appreciated all of her Bockiness. Except that, as I stared, the evening light shifted just a bit: Think of how clouds pass over a field and change the light on the grass. And with this shift, what jumped out at me were bits and pieces of her mother: the complexion so pale as to almost be transparent, the wild field of freckles blooming on her cheeks, the outlines of blue veins visible beneath the transparent, freckled skin near her temples.

My daughter appeared impossibly beautiful. Profoundly innocent. The kind of innocence that inspires, unlocking kindness in the human soul. One of those moments a parent knows he needs to cherish, appreciate. Maybe I needed to be getting the camera on my phone?

Except that by thinking about getting my phone, I wasn't staying in the moment, but instead was concerning myself with an action that was, sorta, the opposite of appreciation.

Her jawline—square then pointed, also like her mom's—was set, her front teeth clenched. Beneath her chin, her violin was trembling a little.

"Can I stop," Lily asked. "My neck hurts."

In the window, snow fell steadily, the day's natural light all but disappeared.

"Almost done," I said.

FACT: ANY SCHMO can small talk at a dinner party, make a good impression for thirty minutes—hell, even an hour. It's after dessert has been cleared, after that refill of a good white, after the A material and trusted anecdotes have been trotted out and someone's gotten comfortable and let their guard down a bit—that's when you learn who has to opine about things they clearly know zero about, who enjoys talk of sedition and racial jokes, who's the bouncing psycho with an ego that cannot be contained. That's when true nature is revealed.

Six weeks in, say. Scarves were being wrapped around necks with dutiful care. Leaves were clogging drainage gutters. Literally *everyone* was getting over the fall bug that had been going around. Lily hadn't remained all that keen on her instrument or her promises. On the plus side, she'd had her first afterschool playdate. (Imagine long stretches of two fun, happy girls—as well as crying bursts about who got to play with the Dorothy/Wicked Witch doll.) We'd shared untold walks home from school, during which I'd been filled in on what letters they learned about. We'd adapted the "Clean Up, Clean Up" song as a catchall tune that could have its lyrics altered for almost any purpose. Lily also had done well at her first away game—that is, her first visit to a friend's house without me staying—though it's also true that at dinnertime, the mom had called to mention Lily getting scared and panicky about new food.

Sure, there had been one or two birthday party meltdowns, although when that much sugar was involved, who didn't freak? Nothing out of the ordinary.

I arrived at the courtyard. Her two teachers took me aside.

"There might be some socialization issues," one said. The other added, "We've had to talk to her, just a few times, for being bossy to her table friends."

Three days later, Lily had a tantrum during recess. "She wanted to dictate, make the game rules for everyone."

I answered that I watched other children needing to have their own way in the courtyard. "I see other kids melting down after they're told 'No.'"

"We all see those things," the brunette teacher said. "It's normal for the age."

"You're telling me Lily's outbursts are necessarily *worse*?"

They waited me out. "We understand that she's been through a lot."

"YOU CAN'T RUIN this child," Dr. Jennifer Melfi assured me.

Cinnamon gummy hearts were fused into the inside front pocket of my jeans, left over from February, most likely. We were in that stretch when you think you're finally done with thermal underwear. I made a mental note about getting spring clothing out of its bin.

Her office. One of our intermittent reviews: checking in on Lily's progress, my concerns.

"Is it so unusual to not be Mozart?" Melfi asked. "Do you think little Wolfgang could actually hold his violin right when he was three?"

I finished wrestling off my sweater, discarding it on the other side of the couch.

I was sitting on the edge, rocked in place, and stopped. "Remember you told me Lily said she was the doll who could do no right?"

Melfi paused, her forehead pointing toward me.

"Okay, so, irrespective of me, putting aside my untold negative influences on her: Is it possible, somewhere deep inside, Lily believes she can't do anything right? That she *deserves* negative attention?"

"You think Lily blames herself for her mother's death?" Melfi asked.

I ran my hand over my forehead. "Saying it out loud, it sounds fucking dark." I tugged my earlobe. "Way too much there to get to in an hour."

"Thirty-eight minutes, actually."

"Smaller bites, then," I said. "What I *can* worry about, I keep seeing her doing okay—following directions, you know, for a little. Then she arrives. That split in the road."

"I'm not sure I know what you mean."

"All right. This girl from my high school? She wasn't singularly bright or particularly creative. But she volunteered for every club, studied her retinas out, every quiz."

Melfi twirled a pen, seemed like she was following.

"I wanted a future but was afraid, I thought I wasn't good enough. So I sat in the back of classes and fucked off and was sarcastic. This girl was determined. She ended up on scholarship to an Ivy."

"You want Lily to be like her."

"Not just to be able to do things. To *want* to learn how to do them."

"Lily's not even four years old."

"Right," I said.

"She's still in a primal place, Charles."

I felt myself get excited, resumed my rocking on the couch's edge. "It's just that first moment where she gets rattled. Where things don't go well and now she's faced with choices. How bad does she want to do this? Does she really want to be shown? Is there any chance of her sticking with a difficult task by herself?"

Dr. Melfi asked, "You don't think you're jumping the gun?"

"Maybe I am. But one of the things I want least in this world is for her fears to grow roots."

"Charles, push her like this, I promise, each time you want her to do something—"

"I don't want her inability to pay attention to become foundational."

"—she'll stop being interested. The second she knows you want it, she'll stop."

"But—"

"You don't have to ascribe it to blaming herself for her mother's death." Jennifer Melfi's voice was firm. "But she *is* missing her mother. Can't you see she's overwhelmed?"

"Right."

"Be patient. Give yourself a break."

For the first time, I leaned back. "Yeah."

"Give *Lily* a break." With enough force that meant she needed to be heard, Dr. Melfi repeated: "You are *not* going to ruin this child."

A TUESDAY AFTERNOON, meaning I had to hustle over from the undergrad class I'd started teaching. Arriving at the Third Street courtyard a few minutes behind schedule, I was harried, as usual, sweating pretty good, my hoodie pocket stuffed with seaweed snacks: Let's hope today I grabbed a package of regular flavor from the bodega, and not wasabi.

When I got to the courtyard, Lily was busy with a group of kids. Actually, she was breaking off from the group.

I watched my child's attention pivot—toward one of the mothers. A creative director (stylish, wedding rock as big as the Ritz, take-no-shit attitude). This woman had shown kindness to Lily in the past weeks, making sure to first get a nod from me, delivering a fresh strawberry into Lily's cupped hands, offering a spritz of bug spray.

Presently, Lily's face was warning-light red. She was paying attention to what Creative Director Mom was saying.

"What's going on?" Heading over, I tried to keep my voice even. "Everything all right?"

"She gave it to me." Lily kept her hands behind her back.

"It's mine," went the other girl.

"It's her hair clip," Creative Director explained. From her expression, I saw she'd tired of Lily's exploits. "We bought it over the weekend."

Obviously, the clip belonged to the other girl. This was a chance to be firm yet empathetic, establish a pattern of the larger good being most important.

Lily was adamant, in full waterworks mode. *"It's not FAIR."*

"Is there anything . . . ?" I said to the mother. "Maybe Lily could have it tonight? We'd bring it back tomorrow?"

Creative Mom looked confused. "I don't think that would be right."

Taking Lily aside, I said, "We'll go shopping. I know a row of stores. We can find you a pretty vintage clip of your own."

Lily jerked away, let out something piercing.

"Sweetie," I said.

She dug in, bawled that much harder.

When she'd been upset as a baby, more than once Diana told me, "Let her cry." Rocking her toward calm, Diana would tell Lily,

"Go ahead, girl, it's all right. Express yourself. Take as long as you need."

"Can you calm down?" I questioned myself as much as her, ordered as much as asked.

Wiping away her snot bubble, I continued. An exhaling breath. "Lily, my love?"

She looked to me. Hopeful. I was on her team.

"Would you please give the clip back?"

Lily twisted out of my grasp. She kept her fist clenched around the clip, held it away from me, flailed, cried out again.

Common sense suggests heads turned. This was a distraction. The mothers looked a few seconds. That was that.

But I felt their acute attention, became convinced of their gawking—all the moms who'd been cool enough, but really never had trusted my gender to begin with, the ones who'd clocked my snide remarks, my aura of disgruntled servitude, how I implicitly judged them, the life paths they'd chosen, the mothers who worried I had an ulterior motive for showing up every day in that courtyard, that maybe I was prowling for bored moms to bed. All of these mothers were staring bullets.

And not just them—those few acquaintances I always sat close to and conversed with, kind women who offered playdates for Lily with their kids, who at least gave me some props for the effort I put in every day but who also saw that, realistically, my daughter needed help. They were watching me, too, keeping their distance, leaving me alone to deal.

"ENOUGH," I said. "LILY."

She stopped kicking my shin, stopped squirming in my grip. Her expression was still frenetic, fire through her cheeks and eyes, the gap of her open mouth. Now Lily zeroed in on me, focusing, squinting. She closed her mouth, set her jaw. Stillness took her. My daughter appeared possessed, taken by a sense of herself—no, by more than that. I recognized this—every bit of the misery I felt. One of my legendary shitty expressions, manifest on my little girl. Only Lily wasn't just channeling my misery; she was claiming it, remixing it. Eyes electric, she was directing my misery back, *toward me.*

THERE THEY WERE, all my worst inner conflicts, not just on display in that courtyard but coming home to roost. I was indeed the one being exposed, once again Bocking things up. And the thing is, it's not like you just recognize the problem, clap your hands, and, *clap clap*, everything gets better. Lily showed up to school the next day. She had some standout moments in class, some stumbles, and then, that afternoon, I picked her up. Playdates took place, friendships melted down, quickly recovered just fine, or maybe opened a breach. Whether my unintentional influence was the direct cause, whether the deeper issues connected with her missing a mother were coming to the fore, ratios of how much of this, proportions of that, the answers were most definitely *not* apparent. Time moved in the only direction it knows. We stumbled along in its gale, trying to plant our feet here, get some leverage there, and then, pretty much the same way that one of Hemingway's characters famously went broke— "gradually and then suddenly"—her fourth birthday approached. Meaning, the first anniversary of Diana's death. Lily and I had been through a full year of this. *A year.*

If anyone deserved a celebration, it was this child. I brought cupcakes to school for all the little lovies. Even better, a friend's wife called. She'd procured us tickets to *Mary Poppins* on Broadway.

A week before the show, I explained: "We have to prepare. That means a moratorium goes into effect."

Lily stared at me, then the computer screen.

No more Natalie Wood lip-synching to Marni Nixon?

No Liesl dancing around the arboretum with that Nazi?

She looked upset, did not understand.

"From here on," I said, typing into the YouTube search engine, "we're full-on supercalifragilistic. All the expialidocious."

That fancy blue dress fit her better than ever, God bless it. Lily looked radiant. We arrived at the theater super early, immediately dropping an heiress's ransom—more cash up in flames—at the merch table, netting ourselves candy, a dolly, a child's tee, a flying umbrella. One more example of so many of us around her—*me*, first and foremost—trying to buy away the pain, to provide her with something fantastic that could not be availed in her real life? And of all possible shows, *Mary Poppins!* The story of a woman magically flying down from the clouds to tend for children and make this broken family all better!

Reader, it surely was overcompensating. Sign me the fuck up.

The usher handed us Playbills; we headed down the aisle, admiring the hall's gilded ornaments, its elegant balconies. I'd spent my life getting discount tickets, heading up to the nosebleeds. These seats weren't just good; they were right in the middle of the orchestra, and as we waded into the sea of tourist parents and their exceedingly cute daughters—of course wearing sequined outfits—I could not help but wonder about the coinage that must have been dropped for these tickets. How could I ever properly thank these people?

Arriving at our seats, unwrapping from our coats. Lily and a nearby girl started talking, and fed off one another's excitement, and soon were looking through their programs, pointing. I stored our swag, collapsed into my seat, felt a rush of relief, high-fiving myself for getting her here.

For a few moments I watched Lily, just looking at her: talking, animated, engaged.

The announcement came from overhead concerning phones and candy wrappers. The lights dimmed. I felt Lily's body tense.

I tensed as well. She'd experienced all of one movie theater in her young life. How could I have overlooked the traumatic event that was lights turning off inside a huge hall?

And I'd prepped her for live music, right?

The orchestra began their slow pound toward the show's overture. On cue, Lily screamed.

"It's all right." I leaned over. *"It's part of the show."*

Her mouth widened so I could see deep to her tonsils. She wailed louder.

The music's pace increased; Lily kept bawling. Whatever I tried, it was obvious her cries were not about to end.

Now, from behind a fluorescent beam of flashlight spotlighted my child, the usher leaned toward me, his whisper directing us.

Lily's face was fully crimson and her mouth was wide and I was gathering up all our merch, making jerking motions, rising in a crouch and taking her hand. I was easing us between the other parents and kids on our row, "Sorry ... Excuse us ... Sorry."

Our walk of shame ended; we emerged into the lights of the lobby. The usher firmly, if politely explained we couldn't be allowed back inside while Lily was a distraction to the other guests.

I crouched. "Take breaths."

Then I followed my own instructions, breathing out.

We could take as long as we needed, said the usher.

Lily sniffed. She looked at me with those saucerlike watering eyes.

"Daddy," she said.

I knew from her tone. She wanted to go home.

"Don't you want to see 'A Spoonful of Sugar'?" I asked.

"Daddy."

I have previously mentioned the male capacity to feel sorry for himself, how easy it is to take that first step. I was now slaloming, in full plummet.

December's air was crisp on our faces. Side by side, we were heading toward the Times Square subway station. A hard pulse rocked my temples, throbbed through my neck.

Philip Seymour Hoffman had been on Broadway that spring for seventy-eight performances of *Death of a Salesman*. I sure hadn't been able to see that.

Hadn't even *thought* about tickets to see Pacino in the thirtieth-anniversary remounting of *Glengarry Glen Ross*.

The trip we'd just made . . . the cash we'd incinerated . . . her inability to *just fucking sit there* . . .

And me begging—*on my knees*—for us to stay, to watch that reductive, soul-sucking Disney-fied bullshit.

Sharp pain down the middle of my forehead; something inside me cracking open.

All my friends, all the nannies and sitters, the teachers, the therapists, both mine and hers, the money, the institutions, the entirety of this jury-rigged support network, a literal year spent building it, propping it up, thinking and researching and sweating, learning in advance potential dangers, mapping the danger zones, meeting the enemy, knowing it was them, it was us, defusing all bombs, blowing ourselves to smithereens, anything anyone could imagine, create, borrow, purchase, steal—

And still a lifetime to be spent outside the ballet, waiting for the doors to open.

A lifetime alone in the park, watching rich, healthy Shake Shack parents who had no clue.

Once again I'd rammed headfirst into the limitations of best intentions.

Once again I'd exposed, to the light, the stark difference between the ideals of the person I wanted to be and the reality of who I was.

I felt myself giving my life for this little girl, hating the sacrifices but sure as hell making them, busting my ass—*and failing*.

Clearly and definitively failing. Oftentimes. And in the most basic ways.

The single last thing I wanted to do was to make life worse for Lily. Was there any doubt this was happening?

Again I circled back to the big questions, immovable, unavoidable: *What is wrong with me? Why does everything have to be so hard?*

Pedestrians passed us in the other direction; a kindly, aging couple looked us up and down. The man volunteered: "She's a cutie."

"Get fucked," I answered.

We continued homeward. Heading east on Twenty-Third, I noticed Lily lingering, slowing, a few steps behind me. What was wrong now?

Let me tell you.

Having managed to take her doll out of the box on the subway, Lily had become preoccupied, was happily unbuttoning Mary Poppins's blouse.

Nothing was wrong. Not one goddamn thing.

FOUR
YEARS OLD

CHAPTER SIX

From: charles bock <bock███████████@mac.com>
Subject: lily bock withdrawing from violin class
Date: March 25, 2███████████ at 8:43 AM EST
To: ████████████████████████@thirdstreet-musicsch.org

Hey there third street music school. This message concerns Lily Bock. She is enrolled in ████████ ████████'s private violin lesson on Thursday afternoons, and the group class on Friday.

Lily is withdrawing from the class, effective immediately.

Two of the three March sessions were canceled on short notice, so we've only had one class in March. You can send me a revised bill for that class. Otherwise we should be fine on the balance.

Thank you for all of your help. I am sure we will take more classes at Third Street. Ms. ███████████ is a wonderful teacher and a lovely lady. In no way is our withdrawing a reflection of her as a teacher,

or her skill, or personality. It is just too hard for me
to get Lily to class and also to practice at home. It's
affecting our relationship in an adverse way and I
think it's better that I find some other activity for
her right now.

Again, I believe her relationship with music will
change as she gets older, and I am sure we will be
around third street more.

Thank you once again for your time.

Charles Bock
Sent via telekinesis.

WINTER'S APEX: AFTERNOON sky the color of filthy snow, Lily off
being educated about how many sides are in a square. I was at my
writing space, not actually writing, not so much, basically distracting
myself, enmeshed in the pleasures of Mark Yarm's *Everyone Loves
Our Town: An Oral History of Grunge*. I was right in the middle of a
chapter, its subject the short-lived, influential Seattle band Mother
Love Bone (members went on to be in Temple of the Dog and
Soundgarden). Their lead singer, Andy Wood, had passed from a
heroin overdose, just a few months before the band's debut album
was going to be released. The singer's significant other—a woman
named Xana La Fuente—was expounding upon her grief, as well as
her subsequent run of sexual partners. La Fuente explained that sex
was part of grief, as sex represented the urge to live.

I read that and had to put down the paperback, its truth resonat-
ing through me: the need to be touched, to be consoled and likewise

soothe, to let loose in a manner that simultaneously brings pleasure and achieves release.

Diana had wanted me to wait a year before dating again. This made sense, in theory. But an abstinent year was a long haul in real time, especially considering my previous two and a half years, which, as you might guess, had been hugely sad and exhausting, and during which—for reasons that also are apparent—I hadn't had any sex. Throw onto that another year, the time following Lily's birth, including the final months of Diana's pregnancy. (Yes, doulas contend that the late pregnancy can be a time when expectant mothers, jacked with hormones, are eager to get down; nonetheless, our home still had not been any kind of cornucopia of erotic offerings.)

I'd survived six months before taking off my wedding ring, replacing it by tattooing, onto my ring finger, the two symbols—an ohm sign and a heart—from the front of Diana's final diary. Another month had passed before I ventured onto a website that not only rated, but provided contact info for sex workers. (Five hundred dollars a pop, the going rate, was both prohibitive and ridiculous.)

Diana and I had married before internet dating took off. Since then, I'd been like every other locked-down, married man on the spinning globe in that I'd followed the rise of this proverbial new Eden from the other side of the plexiglass window. My limited understanding remained that, in this new reality, women had grown empowered and now felt comfortable claiming their orgasms, often while taking selfies. Filthy texts and cock shots weren't just expected, but required elements of courtship. It was every hetero man's fantasy, the pornographic dream that had started as a pubescent and continued throughout adulthood. It might actually be possible to click, meet a girl, have sex, click again, and meet another girl—and that you might endlessly repeat this cycle.

Only we'd moved beyond the realm of fantasy.

Meanwhile, I was firmly in a time of life where you look in the mirror and see deterioration, where a man objectively wonders whether any more real live women will be willing to get naked for him—without a bouncer present—ever again.

I didn't want a girlfriend; that was a no-brainer. I didn't possess the time or mental energy to be seriously interested in anyone. Diana used to indulge all my idiotic rock preferences, my bizarre fandoms; she'd read countless drafts of my doorstop of a novel, showed concern for me if my face was too gaunt, when I was chained too long to my desk without deodorant. She also stepped up, when she had to, and challenged me about my antisocial inclinations, and just how we were supposed to make our way in the real world until the doorstop was finished. No problem getting one of her friends to find me work at a tabloid newspaper. At the end of the night we walked my dog together, watched rented movies on the couch, engaged in the deep conversational good shit that comes with true emotional intimacy. I couldn't imagine the brick-by-brick reconstruction of all that. And as for introducing some imaginary girlfriend for Lily . . .

Real talk: I was nowhere near ready.

All of which is why, amid that winter's festive cornucopia—snow angels with the depth of shallow graves, half-molten snowmen in heroin leans, make-believe friends playing dress-up, sung lyrics to musicals that did not exist—with my body basically rehabilitated and Lily sort of safely accounted for, I apologized to my deceased wife: *so many things* I wished were different. And in the middle of this random weekday afternoon, I typed out the registration info, thereby dipping my figurative toe into the pulsing, virtual cesspool known as AshleyMadison.com, a website whose members were married but were seeking sex outside that marriage. Yeah, Ashley Madison seemed tailor-made for me.

RETURNING FROM A trip to the bathroom; discreetly flipping away from my writing program's window; switching tabs and logging back in—for a discovery. A response. Electricity shot through me. Someone was interested, and not just any someone. Late twenties, looked like. Winking profile, flirtatious. I sent what I hoped was a well-crafted greeting, one that conveyed proper enthusiasm, hopefully even a spark of cleverness: "Okay. Your photos just blew my mind straight through my brain." Within ten minutes I got an answer: "{/:" and followed up, volleyed, worked my way into: Maybe she wanted to chat? "URCute"was her response. "I'm def interested. Only thing. I've had problems w/ stalkers. AshMad won't do anything. For my safety, could you just register at this site." She included a link, apologized for the small sign-up fee. I stopped corresponding, kept getting follow-ups, "*UR so sexy. Just register alreddy so we can have fun.*" At which point I realized: I was not chatting with a person but some kind of bot.

Reader, even *this* felt like progress—maybe not success, not a date, but something happening, or almost happening. Fact is, the greater majority of my attempts had been going straight into the ether, had been ignored, or had been brutally shot down—*by fucking adulterers, of all people.* One time I got catfished and eventually discovered I was dealing with an online prostitute, a woman who was obviously insane, on meth, and out of my price range. This still didn't stop me: I was a starving man in a dumpster, and though I didn't make an appointment with the overpriced catfish, I nonetheless kept on dumpster diving, adjusting my profile in between tough paragraphs at my writing space, sending texts while watching the kid attempt backbends in her courtyard.

An aging party girl kept posting shots of empty Hamptons beaches. She was couch surfing through the offseason; we had a few great chats; I thought I had a shot. In certain terms, she let me know she was looking to land a hedge fund hubby. An executive at a catering service had no problem meeting for afternoon tea. We made out around the corner from her subway stop, but she was not looking to ruin her Upper West Side family, certainly not to risk a fling. (There was no second meeting.) I had lunch with a lovely sad Yemeni woman, in her mid-thirties, whose high-powered husband was never around. During our conversation, I reached beneath the table, touched her stockinged knee, and pressed. The flash that took her, that connected us, was tangible, her desire suddenly electric. She was exotic, a platinum blonde, dark skinned. She wore a prim white jacket. Her face was just as it had been five seconds earlier; at the same time, it was transformed, near tears, simultaneously frightened and so erotic as to be paralyzing. We still had our orders coming. Neither of us knew what was next. We kept chatting. By the time our meal ended, it was clear the moment had passed, her desires were going to stay bottled—at least, with me.

A nice woman was stuck on Long Island, trapped in an open marriage. She'd rather have been locked down and happy, and she was pissed at Hubby, looking for retribution. We exchanged a few emails, ended up walking along the High Line. Oblivious to the chilled afternoon, I asked if she wanted ice cream. (A go-to move. One of my friend's teen years had been spent pulling tourists in a rickshaw around the beaches of Oahu, Hawaii. Afterward, he'd tell the single women he knew where to get the best ice cream on the island.) Ice cream was innocent, reaching back into childhood. Ice cream also was creamy, melting on the tongue.

I bought this lovely unhappy woman a cup of chocolate mint and talked her into going to the last hourly hotel in Chelsea. Our kisses were heated. My first time having sex since my marriage. Every second felt foreign, wrong, and at the same time sacred. Afterwards, she sent an affectionate email. I replied with warmth. That was the only time we met.

LOOKING BACK, I see that I worked hard to listen to Dr. Melfi's assurance: "You cannot ruin this child." I tried to take value in her words, to will her truth into action, in one breath fretting, cursing, clenching my fists until my knuckles were white; in the next, believing in Lily's strength, unclenching, breathing, letting our lives just move forward without eruption, with something that might have resembled faith.

Daddy wiped under his daughter's fingernails to get out all of the watercolor paint. When Lily turned without a second thought, Daddy watched her trot away, toward new fun. Daddy picked up the glass of dirty water, wiped paint off the table surface.

Daddy stood outside the woman's bathroom at the puppet show, apologized to a woman who was on her way in. "Could you do me a favor? Just check on my daughter. Her name is Lily."

"No, Daddy cannot come and help play with your dollies right now," I said. "He has to keep lying on the couch to keep it from flying up to the ceiling."

Lily, delighted: *"Daddy, the couch does not fly."*

Lily shouting out Muppet gibberish with me, rolling balls of cookie dough for the oven pan. Here she was, standing on my feet at the edge of our little kitchen, the two of us contradicting each other over whose turn it was to lick the remains of the frosting mix from off the bowl. (I will spare you any suspense: it was always her turn.)

Then she was in our bathroom, finishing on the potty, and was playing, unspooling the toilet paper roll, and somehow locked herself in, and I had to put my shoulder through the flimsy door, and Lily screamed and cried. Who wouldn't?

We were in the West Village playground, near my sister's apartment. Lily had her legs hooked on the bottom rung of some protective fence bars; she was hanging on to the top bars, and for no discernible reason decided to let go. I was sitting, like, six inches away on a bench, and actually saw this happen, her actions making no sense to me, disagreeing with all logic, I even had enough time to think, *What are you*— Then her head plummeted, and the rest of her body followed along, swinging as if on a hinge, the back of her skull banging against the pavement, its impact sickening. In the emergency room specifically for children, we were put through to an exam room, and as we waited for a doctor, gradually Lily's howls petered out into whimpers, and her whimpers ebbed and then picked back up, a bit, and she swung a little bit around on the doctor's chair, and I helped her climb up onto the exam table, and she crinkled the thin paper, and since the room was legit frigid, I found a blanket, and she wrapped herself like a little burrito. When I was done with my half-hearted attempt to eat her face, I took out whatever coins I had, explaining the value of pennies, nickels, dimes, quarters. An hour or so like that, minimum progress on the money front, but wasn't that part of it, the point of these waiting rooms—especially when it's not a life-or-death situation— the boredom, taking the edge off, seeping away at her fear? And when it came time for her sutures, Lily followed my instructions, shut her eyes, reached for the safety of my hand, gave a big, hard squeeze.

But we also had my longtime friend Terri Jay Cello dropping in, purchasing not one but two full-length puffy winter coats for

Lily! We had another buddy, Kashmir, hauling his kids to our house and forcing them to act out scenes from *The Sound of Music* with her! That well-meaning married couple from my writing space who started popping in for Saturday night visits, doing a kind of soft rehearsal for their own attempts at parenting, whisking Lily off to a coffee shop for burgers and board games and ice cream! Another guy I'd traded sarcasms with on a long-ago part-time job welcomed us into his home for dinner! Still another writer, cleaning her closet, sent packages of clothes her daughter had outgrown! What basically amounted to reinforcements, thank the Flying Spaghetti Monster for these good people, and more than I can list here: they kept me from blowing my brains out, seriously they did. And, reader, it is no exaggeration to say, I resented every single one of those motherfuckers.

A YOUNGISH BARISTA met me at some other ice cream parlor in the West Village. Underneath slovenly clothes she hid the promise of legendary breasts. She had been a chess prodigy, competitive into her teen years, but still wasn't recovered from flaming out, and was on so much depression medication that she could not come. I took this explanation as a challenge, and tried to conquer science by lifting her atop a chest of drawers. The wooden fixture banged repeatedly against the walls of our cheap art hotel; afterward, she asked if we could start having lunches. Eat good food. Maybe *talk* before our trysts.

That was it for her.

SEX WAS A significant part of what these women were searching for. I see this now. I also understand they had not been receiving emotional intimacy from their husbands, no exciting sparks from the people in their lives, no needed embraces from the outside world. Ashley Madison promised they could be wanted, mooned over, valued as womanly, sexual beings without throwing away the lives they'd built. And they also got to embark on something new, which is always a thrill—to define (or redefine) themselves for someone new, to flirt, be worthwhile in new eyes, explore new attractions: they got a *secret*.

Granted, recognizing all this, especially in retrospect, is not quantum physics. Still, when it was happening, if you'd read those previous sentences to me, I would have nodded, *Right*. Then, boom, emotional intimacy would have been one more tool, something I had to provide, promise, or feign. "The secret of success is sincerity," goes the famed quote attributed to forgotten playwright Jean Giraudoux. "Once you can fake that, you've got it made."

A close friend once confided that, during stretches of life where she was having sex, she walked differently than if she wasn't. Her statement acknowledges the innate. You just feel better when you're getting off, when you're getting someone else off.

As for responsibility for fostering those emotional attachments? Owning up to any expectations I'd nurtured? I didn't have the emotional space. Lily dominated my radar screen.

That is what I told myself.

AS IF ON cue:

"I want to grind," she said.

"You can't grind," I answered.

"But I want to grind."

My little girl, my Lilisita Mon Amita, positioned against the corner of the small white table that acted as her desk, was thrusting without compunction or self-consciousness. Two feet away, her godmother stared, slack-jawed. Over to take Lily out for dinner, Susannah had been chitchatting with me about how much she didn't enjoy a particular consulting job. Eyes then went wide, the conversation stopping.

A child's sexuality is a delicate subject, obviously. But wasn't it supposed to be her teen years that this minefield would detonate, exploding upon both Lily and me?

To have this now? Really?

Susannah mumbled something. I started punching at my phone. Parenting sites agreed: grinding was appropriate for a girl that age.

"Go in the bedroom if you need to."

Lily dutifully dismounted, scampered off.

I looked at Susannah, shrugged. *What am I supposed to do?*

I WAS SUPPOSED to apply enough attention, insight, and precision to my edits of fifteen homework essays that my intermediate fiction students would be able to unlock the myriad nuclear truths that lay inside those dormant passages. I was supposed to be firm with the pesky creditor and convey that what they had labeled a *generous offer*—me paying thirty cents on the dollar—was mistaken, as my name, in fact, had *not* been on Diana's grad school health insurance policy, meaning I was *not* legally responsible for the expenses on the bills they kept hounding me about, so they could go inhale a big bag of walrus asshole. I was supposed to get stamps, send out checks, keep good shit like electricity from being disconnected. I was supposed to return a weird query about teaching a graduate-level workshop online. Make up a blurb for a book I gave up on around chapter three. I was supposed to get to the Fourteenth

Street Trader Joe's for groceries during that twenty-three-minute sweet spot that exists right after the senior citizens have done their weekly shopping but before the college kids have woken up and figured out they need supplies for their weekend. Handle paperwork for Lily's pre-K field trip on the Staten Island Ferry. Send an email to my therapist with my insurer's out-of-network code for psychological services. I was supposed to finally check in on my parents and then call my sister back to let her know I'd done as much. Scale to level four of Laundry Mountain. Lily was at Third Street, so the onus was on me.

Whatever else I was supposed to be doing, it was also unavoidably true: if I wasn't heading toward the page count that got me the next installment of my advance, then I was moving us toward bankruptcy, toward homelessness. It weighed on me. Even meeting friends for lunch felt sketchy.

Unless, of course, it was Terri Jay Cello.

We'd met at an arts colony—I'd been working on my first book, she'd taken a leave from her office gig to finish an orchestral composition—and through this past, Jesus, this past *decade*, her benevolence toward me had been, by any rational account, astonishing. It had started with her illegally subletting that Gramercy apartment to me after she'd married and moved to Brooklyn. When the management company discovered our deception and started eviction procedures, Terri Jay convinced them to transfer the lease (telling me, before we all met to sign contracts, "*Don't speak*"). If this wasn't enough, after I'd finished a final draft of my book, Terri Jay snuck me into her place of employment after business hours and we used their printers, Xeroxed the manuscript, and sent the copies off to agents. She was one of the people who helped organize a fundraiser that absorbed Diana's medical costs, was bedside with Diana during those last days. Basically, Terri Jay Cello was my guardian angel, one of the few people I felt safe with, to whom I could confide without reservation.

That afternoon, Terri had a rehearsal but suggested coffee, and though I didn't drink coffee, she insisted, even volunteering to schlep her instrument all the way downtown.

We were at an upscale spot not all that far from my writing space. A table in back, next to a busboy folding napkins, stacking them onto a catering cart.

Nibbling on a complicated scone, Terri Jay listened to and at the same time seemed to be studying me, tracking something about my shirt. Her napkin went to my water glass, dabbed at my chest bone, its blemish of soy sauce. She smiled, a bit amused.

"A lot of what you're describing sounds pretty normal," she said. "To me, anyway."

"Oh," I said. "We're fucked beyond words."

Her response was nonplussed, her expression staying placid, but in a way that somehow seemed to harden her. A good ten years older than me, her face still retained its classic, almost Grecian bone structure, its pristine beauty. Terri had always known things, always had appeared to be knowing, but she had a different, deeper depth now, the years adding unavoidable gravitas, an integrity that could not be impugned.

"Not—" I waved my napkin. "I mean, Lily's a handful, but a great handful." Eye contact. Something in me wanted to get out. Did I even know what I was getting at, how to make myself known? I kept trying. "Sometimes it's just a lot, you know?"

"It *is* a lot." Terri Jay set her hands in front of her. "But Lily's such a fun little adventurer. I'm sure all kinds of good things are happening."

Her goodwill was genuine. That smile so kind, almost letting me off the hook. Reminding me of my indebtedness. The neon sign, suspended over me, buzzing, blinking: *Step in, save us.*

"You were nice to volunteer to come down here," I said. "Especially seeing that you have to drag that giant instrument."

Terri Jay reached for my hand. "It's my pleasure."

"Everyone's so nice like that, happy to check in on me. 'Is Charles washing dishes? Is Charles keeping up the apartment?'"

Her hand stopped. I continued:

"'Does Lily have clothes. Is Lily still breathing?'"

Keeping eye contact, Terri blinked, doing so in a manner that had specific purpose, a calming blink, a blink designed to clear this slate. She waited a count. "What about your private life? Are you getting out at all?"

"Honest? I get a break." One at a time my fingers shot out: "Exhaustion. Relief."

"Charles, I'm sure there are good—"

"Oh, definitely Terri. There are."

"Charles."

"What? You want the lowdown on my kamikaze wife fuck sessions down by the West Side Highway?"

That did it: her eyes bulged, her expression twisting, mouth dropping. Now Terri's hand became a fist; that fist strangled her napkin.

"This is the best I can do, Terri." I kept going. "Maybe that's the worst of it, how bad my best ends up being."

Her eyes trembled at the edges. She did not look away. She said my name again, but the way she spoke this time—*"Charles,"* soft, defeated—hit me.

"What's wrong with you?" Terri asked.

And now, looking at the fragile woman across the table, I realized information I already well knew: Terri Jay Cello had tried for years to have kids—with her husband and also through science. All the efforts she'd made, everything I was saying—I saw their reverberations, all playing out across her face.

But I saw something else too.

ALL THAT AFTERNOON, my guardian angel's expression tightened around my throat. Returning to my writing cubicle wasn't an option. I needed to walk through my discomfort, and so I wandered the teeming streets of downtown. Hipsters were staring at their phones, busy with their texts, or whatever it is that keeps them from looking out straight in front of them. I almost knocked into a few, felt an urge to mow through them, felt uncertain of my destination, nonetheless eager to reach it.

Terri had been afraid. This was the thing I had to come to terms with. And her fear had not been for me. In no way was her concern for my benefit.

There was someone far more important to be worried about.

Finally, I arrived up at the aptly named Books of Wonder, the only store in the city fully devoted to children's books.

"We're going to solve this bullshit."

"Sir?" The clerk glanced around, maybe looking for security.

"Yeah. Could you look up any books for toddlers with these words in the title."

Waiting, making sure the clerk was ready. "'Wart.' 'Toon.' 'Leaf,' and—right—'*egg*.'"

A tentative nod, typing.

"Maybe she jumbled them," I said. "Add 'heart.' 'Tin.'"

Polite, uncomfortable seconds passed. I might have called the clerk Galadriel. May have explained that Galadriel was the lady of light who helped Frodo on his quest. As the clerk led me into the aisles, I may or may not have apologized for my cursing. I may or may not have said the weird Tolkien reference was just to lighten the mood. I may have admitted it was a misguided attempt, one bad thing after another, and then thanked the clerk for doing me a solid. I may or may have not explained that I needed something to make my little girl happy, may or may not have let the clerk guide me to the toddler section, then rush the hell away, back to the front counter.

Fun fact: children's shelves are built for the eye levels of kiddies, not those of parents. I felt things crackling through my knee and lower back, but knelt down and started reading spines.

At bedtime, I rushed Lily into her jammies, let her skimp on the teeth brushing, urging her forward. The moment of truth arrived: from the pile on the floor, I unveiled a specific hardback, its new cover shining forest green.

Lily stopped climbing on my shoulder and neck. She halted all of her tricks to delay bedtime.

Staring at the cartoon image on the cover, she listened to my instructions. Settling now into my side, she half pushed both feet against my arm, using it as leverage. She pulled on my earlobe, enjoying its flexibility.

I flipped to the title page, announced a title.

All pulls ended. Her voice was bright: "The Horton story?"

Hands to her mouth, light emanating her face.

At long last.

Horton Hatches the Egg. The story where the mother takes off and the elephant has to sit on the eggs.

The grin on her face remained a revelation.

On one level, it was true, I just hadn't known the name of *whatever* that Elefegg title had been.

There also was another level. This particular book. I'd actually been staying away from it.

The fact is, Lily had already heard *Horton Hatches the Egg*. The day after Diana's death. A gentle woman—Diana used to do spa massages with her in SoHo—was trying to help, giving me a break. When I returned with groceries, the woman was ghost white, apologetic. Lily had asked for the book. The woman hadn't known what to do.

"You tell her NO," I'd said. "You're the ADULT."

I'd thrown out that old copy. But you bet your ass, Lily'd remembered, she had *desired* this story, trying to sound out its title to her parade of sitters, asking me for her version of the title when she was scared, when she was nervous, the night before school started. Had they read it at Third Street?

I found the starting page. "Okay."

Lily focused on each new illustration like a general receiving access to enemy plans. She similarly excelled at turning pages at *just* the right moment.

She inhaled that story. *Devoured* it.

To her that elephant was the *real parent*.

Twisting in place beneath the comforter, Lily *celebrated* that elephant.

And when the mommy bird returned, Lily was every bit as thrilled.

"I want Horton to stay in the nest with the mommy bird."

Somewhere a plane was taking off. Somewhere a universe was being born.

Lily kept sitting up, those eyes waiting for my answer. Her solution seemed natural. Why was I taking so long to tell her the logical next step?

What could I say?

Whenever I'd thought about the story, the truth is, I'd fixated on the fact that Maizey, the dilettante mommy bird, had chosen to take flight, abandoning her daughter just so she could snort rails with the band. Meanwhile, in real life, Diana. It pissed the shit out of me. And now here we were, Lily explaining it to me again: "The mommy bird and Horton can take care of the baby together."

I looked at her, felt wonder, felt more than I could even process.

And recognized something. Plugging into it now. Finally.

The schism.

Could I get beyond grimy daily mechanics, stop feeling sorry for myself long enough to just, you know, *experience* this little girl next to me?

Could I feel the value—in her, in this: taking care of my child, yes, but also all the residuals—emotional strength, stability, warmth—that came with being loved by her?

I'd been able to find the Horton book, yes. But *being* Horton, in all his Hortonness—was I honestly up to the challenge?

Because it was obvious, this child was desperate.

Like the way she always straightened up and listened close at the beginning of *Cinderella*, going still for that part where the mom dies, her eyes concentrating on those pages while Ella's dad remarries.

Lily *wanted* to hear those stepsisters ragging on Cinderella. Was *ravenous* to watch those family dynamics play out.

A sense of awe had me: the completeness, the magnitude, of my child's desire.

Here she was, searching every cloud.

CHAPTER SEVEN

Dear Charles,

If I die in the next little while, I am afraid that you will let your darkness take over your personality. I just want you to know that I hope with all my heart that you will fight that eventually and not stay there. You can have a wonderful life without me. You can meet someone else who can be a good partner for you, a good mom to Lily. But that will only work if you open yourself to that possibility. If I die I will be an angel looking after you, putting the right person in your life, trying to help you however I can from the other side. Have faith in me. Have faith in my love for you, my desire for your happiness. We have so much to celebrate, so much love, so many amazing experiences together. If it all ends sooner than we want, that doesn't mean you can't be happy again. I will give you a year to mourn, and then I will start working for your joy. I'm more worried about you being OK than Lily. And I'd be less worried about her when I think about you getting back on your feet and moving forward with your life after I'm gone.

Right now you are the best partner anyone could ask for. You bring me so much joy and warmth and nurturing. I want to spend years with you as a healthy person, enjoying our connection and savoring this incredible bond we have, going through hell together as we have been. I want to co-parent with you and share that adventure.

If I don't get to do that, I don't want you to do it alone. I encourage you to be open to love. Be open to goodness. You deserve every happiness, and if I can't be here to help fill your life with joy, then I really want you to find someone almost as wonderful as me who can be a great partner for you. People do this. They move on. You will. Wait a year, and then be back in the world fully. If my version of the universe is right, I will be helping from the other side.

You are such a source of joy and comfort for me. Thank you for everything. I love you.

THE ONSET OF summer, or thereabouts. Two women entered my life, pretty much at the same time. Their joint appearances set into motion events that, let's say, uh, *accelerated* a certain unavoidable confrontation. and this *mishegas* forced me to address an issue that I quite honestly did not want to deal with, questions I had no intention of asking of myself. What, basically, amounted to potential ruin for me and my daughter.

So, yeah. A lot to unpack.

Stealing the words of Julie Andrews: Let's start at the very beginning.

An invitation, a film screening. Like, once every nine months I got one, usually at random, some tangential connection, a favor, a friend who couldn't use the tickets. Tonight's show was an independent film, the adaptation of a legendary novel—exactly the kind of juxtaposition that results in either profound success or rollicking disaster.

On the end of the back row, in a half-empty screening room, I passed time before the lights dimmed, marking up pieces for class. A few seats to my left, a pair of fashiony, extremely hip women were having a great time, entertaining each other: the farthest one shut her eyes and leaned her head back, unleashing a deep laugh, all but howling at the moon. Meanwhile, the nearer one kept talking, rolling her wrist, gesturing with her hand, basking in this ridiculous story she was unfurling. These women were obviously fun, sharp, and easy to stare at, especially when the one nearest me (princess ringlets, oversized shades) dove into her purse. Hearing the emergent ringtone—the chorus of a popular hip-hop song—I was surprised.

"I didn't know phones could have songs as their ringtones," I managed.

The close one seemed to have heard me, her body language responding enough for me to continue, my voice going firm. "Me and my inconsistent ballpoint feel out-of-date."

She took her time, gave me a once-over. "Did you just say your ballpoint's impotent?"

"It's tragic. You'd never guess, but this pen? In its heyday, a *stallion*."

She almost smirked. Soon enough she was volunteering that she was a stylist, ran down clothes for magazine shoots. I scribbled her name in my homework folder so I wouldn't forget. Let's call her Z.

Days later, at the writing space, I mentioned her name to an acquaintance, a woman who freelanced for different fashion magazines and, as such, knew a web of media players. My acquaintance smiled—too wide?—and agreed to check about forwarding contact info. Days passed. Maybe Z said no? Was my acquaintance subtly waving a red flag: *Ease away from this one?*

I ignored the possibility, asked her again.

Little did I suspect this script was about to complicate: an email. Popping into my inbox. Subject: *Been a while.*

Let's call our new entrant A. Publicist from the West Coast. Wiry and caustic, piercing green eyes, crafted Midwestern features, most of which ended in sharp angles. We'd met when my novel had come out. During a few professional conversations, there had been sparring, even a spark, maybe a sense that, in a different life, things might have lined up. In this life, however, I already was married. A also had gotten married, and Lily had been born, and Diana had gotten sick, and, well, we'd fallen out of touch.

A's marriage was over. She was out east. Staying in Queens.

Wait until you are six months into a relationship before introducing any woman to Lily. One of my friends, the writer who sent me boxes of her child's clothing and toys, had been through the dating wars. She dictated the guideline with a finality that left no doubt: she knew what she was talking about.

Of course, being a needy boy-man, I could not listen. The journalist came over one night. Slight, ponytailed, black jeans, thrift store tee. That cute shrewd girl you might see running a merch table for an indie band.

Lily, long accustomed to visitors, easily accepted A, welcoming her to the little white worktable. "Do you want to make princesses," she asked.

A's expertise was in massaging reporters and their questions, keeping backstage feuds out of the public. Her eyes darted around the living room. "Sure," she answered. Lowering herself to the carpet, she positioned herself in a cross-legged, yogic stance, and picked up the child scissors. "Um, I don't know how to operate these. Do I need a license?"

Lily didn't blanch. A finger, its pads stained by orange marker, pointed. "You have to follow the lines when you cut."

A's work on the princesses was halting, self-conscious. Even in her little yoga pose, her body remained Republican stiff. She kept looking back toward me, wanting some arts-and-crafts relief, hoping to catch up with everything that occurred with my family, attempting, here and there, to volunteer information about the final throes of her own union. Lily cut off her questions, kept her on point.

Once I got Lily down for the night, I asked, "Do you want to stay and talk?"

At some point, the couch happened to fold out.

Breaking away from our kisses, A nodded toward the hallway. "You sure?"

"All the struggle it takes to get her asleep?" I answered. "When she's down, she is down."

A remained skittish. We maintained eye contact with each other. The otherwise silence, the rickety futon, the vibe of clandestine teenagers not wanting to be caught—all became their own turn-ons. Her pupils went large; my hand, covering her mouth, was answered by biting teeth.

But I'd also started seeing Z, the woman with the ringlets, from the screening. It took a bit but my friend did forward her email address, which led to our first meeting, at a dog park, Z and me sitting together while her oversized pug sunned himself atop our picnic table. A second date followed: Sheepshead Bay, old-school French-dip sandwiches. For each outing, she flashed bling, wore different, noticeably oversized eyewear. What I remember from those afternoons are her running monologues, her resonant and brackish laughter, arriving at the end of half-hour sentences that twisted around me. I was constantly disentangling myself, trying to get straight on just how she'd hustled up through the ranks of stylists, which celebrity may have been connected to which embarrassing anecdote, bar owners and financiers she'd dated, the big-deal model she no longer spoke with. I was intrigued but also confused, almost a front-row spectator.

Another intricate joke. After considerable build-up, Z took a moment. Batting thick lashes, she snapped the whip on its punch line: *"Lights go on. My friend's like,* Whoa, I'm sucking his arm!"

I was more than happy to laugh.

MEANWHILE, THE SCHOOL year limped into its denouement, and the courtyard mommies had fed on one other's souls pretty thoroughly. Everyone was worn down, myself included. Having reached an unspoken understanding with most of them—*You stay away from me and my kid, we'll stay away from you*—I willfully ignored the various mothers coordinating summer plans to visit one another's second homes, and shouldered the crying jag that resulted after Lily was left out of one too many end-of-the-year pizza picnics.

I folded Lily's summer clothes, underwear, and socks into her miniature suitcase. (*Enough to last a month?* I wondered, remembering there was such a thing as washing machines in Tennessee, stop worrying so much.) I loaded my backpack with snacks, printed out our boarding passes, and then made sure Lily held my hand—not just in the bus station, but while stepping onto the airport escalator. I double-checked that neither of us had left our rolling suitcases in Hudson News.

Among Diana's final wishes was Lily annually spending time with Mom's side of the family, becoming familiar with where her mother came from. Wish granted: the two of us soon touched down in the ailing queen city of Memphis. Lily would visit her grandma for a month. During this time I'd be back in Manhattan. *Thirty days.*

First, though, we walked around in the same riverside park where a teenaged Diana Joy Colbert had loved wasting time. Humidity thick as cake; calliope music drifting from an unseen, docked paddleboat; the mighty Mississippi placid and brown.

A special occasion was on tap for today. Peg wore a neat yellow summer dress and sensible shoes. In one hand she held the strings of a few colored helium balloons. Her other hand lightly clasped Lily's wrist.

Lily bounced up and down. She was wearing the pretty blue frock from her third birthday party, the very same one she'd worn for *Mary Poppins* and for her Third Street school pictures. It still fit, though its hem no longer grazed the ground. Peg had done her hair in blossoming pigtails. Behind the two of them, Diana's beloved aunt Margie and uncle Glenn were unloading, from a sport utility vehicle, what appeared to be a dozen more balloons, corralling them so they did not get away.

Lily could not hold still: she was entranced by the balloons, energized by the sight of the ships along the river, by the park, all the relatives Diana had grown up with—everyone with us, dressed in long dresses, in collared shirts and khakis, each family member with their own balloon.

I watched Lily point at the riverboats, twirl to the calliope melody. I was trailing a few feet behind, letting her and Peg be together. My free hand was rolling my suitcase. In my head, I was back in the exam room, the morning Diana had been diagnosed, watching my infant daughter play with the balloon made from that inflated glove.

Jeez. It really had been a different lifetime.

Peg led us all over rocks, toward the water. Diana, along with her cousins and their circle of friends, used to come out here. Lazy afternoons. Dimming evenings. Boats and port ships slowly going by. They listened to melodic synthesizer music by sad new romantics; they smoked menthols, once in a while tried harder stuff. At that point in her life Diana had won a county spelling bee for which she'd gotten her name into the local paper. She was dreaming about college, getting out of the state, becoming a filmmaker. This would have been before she turned down a scholarship from the local college and enrolled in New York University, well before she became weighed down with college loans and a shitty office job, before she started the wake-and-bake routine that, eventually, would coat the walls and ceiling of her shower in a sticky film of marijuana resin. Diana, her cousins, their friends—they'd been a bunch of teenagers in a park, looking out at the water, talking about music and love and dreams, not even knowing they were inching their way toward the people they'd become.

She and I used to joke that when she was eighty she'd try heroin, because why not? On her deathbed, she had meetings with her Narcotics Anonymous sponsee.

Cloud cover, if any, was faint. A hint of breeze couldn't dent the humidity. I had this feeling that I could reach out and wring the water from the air as if dealing with a wet towel. I wore the same jacket and shirt I'd been married in, felt myself swimming in my own sweat.

The family's procession reached the river's edge. I unzipped my suitcase, removed the red velvet box. From its size it looked as if it might contain a football. I placed the box on the picnic table, undid its two small latches, and removed from it a speckled urn. A faded bluish gray, it looked like something from the time of the Roman Empire.

One of Diana's last wishes had been to release some of her ashes into the Mississippi River, at this rocky bank. But, it turns out, ashes are actually heavy: you're talking about the weight of a human body burned down. Sometimes bone and sinew remain, little chunks. The urn, constructed of a thick marble, felt weighty in my hands, more dense than I'd expected. Its lid took effort to unscrew, but suddenly came loose, *click*.

Lily was running around in circles, trying to climb up a nearby tree. Peg asked her to come over, gave Lily her own balloon to play with.

"Is this an up balloon or a down balloon," Lily asked.

Peg looked confused.

"In *Peppa Pig*, George lets go of an up balloon," Lily said. "Polly Parrot catched up so it did not get away."

"An up balloon," I told Lily.

Each family member read out loud a personal message to Diana, opening a window onto *their* Diana, the girl and woman they'd grown up with: who she'd been, what she'd meant to that person. Each message finished and you understood a little more about loss, how multifaceted it can be, its tones and hues and the many dimensions there can be to our world. And then that reader approached the opened urn; inside it, a plastic bag of industrial thickness contained all of the ashes. Each reader poured out a scoopful, carefully walked the plastic scooper over to the rocks, to the water's lip.

When it was my turn, I mentioned that Diana had been the first person to read my early drafts—and brought that same willing eye to my ninety-eighth drafts. I brought up her good nature, her trying for that grant to give massages to homeless people with AIDS. I talked about the void I felt without her, but also how Diana's love was eminently visible in her daughter, in all of us; we saw it here, in the kindness we showed each other. That was enough speaking for me. Today was for her Memphis family. I wanted to stay out of their way, wanted it all to go well for them.

One at a time, each of us poured some ashes of my late wife's body into the murky water. First the soot piled, then it dissipated. When we were all finished, simultaneously, we released the balloons into the air.

Lily must have sensed this was important, that whatever was happening here somehow related to her. She stopped running, turned her head, watched. Then she took my balloon. Giggling, she let it go, then tried to follow the bunch. Only she could not. Their staggered procession moved horizontally with the slight wind. Single balloons began to separate from one another now, their small circles of color slowly shrinking, drifting over the gray water, toward the gray infinite.

DIANA WENT WITH me to see Slash's solo band. It was early in our dating life, winter, a club on the border of the West Village and Tribeca, and when the venue took extra long to open its doors, Slash came out and walked the line and individually thanked people for waiting out in the cold. A year or so later—we were a couple but still before the marriage—we took a road trip up to Hartford, Connecticut. For that one, there was buzz that Axl's oft-delayed new album might finally be coming out, and he'd gotten his band of talented replacements together, insistently calling them Guns N' Roses. I managed to get us great seats at the Hartford Civic Center. That night, with Axl doing one of his legendary waiting sessions before going on, his camera crew focused on different women in the crowd, continuing a longstanding tradition where the audience encouraged them to flash their breasts, showing them on the arena's Jumbotron. The camera focused on Diana. She sort of laughed. Good luck with that.

The following night, a long-running hard-rock radio show—infamous because its listeners never got stumped by the trivia question, no matter how obscure the metal factoid—was taking calls about Axl and his new band, wanting to know whether listeners would give the new album a chance. I called in and managed to get on the air and pontificate: the old band wasn't getting back together; why not give the new bunch a chance, see what this new material sounds like? When I called Diana to ask what she'd thought, she answered, "I can't talk. I'm on hold to go on the air with him," and clicked on over. She told the host that she'd been at the show and enjoyed watching Guns N' Roses, but she had a problem with how their roving cameras exploited women, and she said that if she paid to go to a rock show, she had the right not to be objectified and treated like a piece of meat. She wanted to know what the host thought of that.

I had been on the ball and taped the entire exchange. We ended up including it—all of it, including the deejay's sputters and hems—as a secret track that we burned onto a CD and included in the goodie bags at our wedding.

One more balloon, shrinking out over the water.

LILY WAS STRAPPED in the booster seat in the rear of the Dodge, watching the scenery outside her window. This passing world was not hers: strip malls, tract housing, shrubbery, the suburbs, unknown for her, exotic, and she was totally into them, her jaw open.

Peg was driving, bringing us into a leafy, pleasant neighborhood of modest single-level homes. Built after the Second World War, each house sat a distance from the curb. In recent years, I knew, limited tax revenues from this zip code had meant cuts to sanitation and essential services. Stories circulated of robbery gangs making the rounds from out of landscaping trucks, seniors holding their wallets close in grocery stores.

The Dodge completed its turn, started down the street. Peg honked, a way to alert the friend who lived a few houses down: *I'm around, just in case.*

"Miss Samantha is so precious." Peggy pointed to her left. "I can't wait for you to meet her."

Lily followed Peg's prompt, peering over.

"My big girl." Peg looked into the rearview mirror. "It's such a blessing to have you here." She smiled at Lily. "We're going to have so much fun." To me she added, "It's a shame Daddy can only stay one day."

I returned her sentiments in kind. Through my front pocket, along my thigh, I could feel my phone's muted pulse: texts. They'd been arriving, on and off, for a while now, likely asking about the ceremony, maybe proposing plans for when I got back to the city. Their possibilities vibrated, pulling at me; I let the phone stay where it was, didn't want to be rude.

Rising out of the front seat, I helped to corral the luggage from the trunk. Peg guided Lily by the hand, led us all toward her home, a neat and cozy little number, brick and clapboard trimmed with blue paint bright and thick as cake icing. She guided us into a living room, where the lights had been left on, a deterrent to anyone who might be casing the place.

Before I could set down any suitcases, well before I could even take in the polite and spotless décor, I was waylaid.

Pictures and portraits lined the walls, filled the bookshelves. It would have been physically impossible to see all of them at once. However, in these moments, I took in more of them than you might think: Diana at fifteen sitting for a profile portrait; Diana in cap and gown, graduating from her high school; a shot of Diana, her mother, and her beloved grandmother, all smiling on a roller coaster; Diana beaming along with me as we entered the reception on our wedding day; Diana embracing Lily seconds after giving birth to her; a thin, post-transplant Diana and baby Lily, smiling, standing together in a garden . . .

I planted my feet, tried to stay solid.

Of course, Lily was mesmerized. After all this time, here was her mother, and from so many angles: Yes, the photos she knew from our home, but new ones, too, everywhere she looked, the experience complete, immersive. Her wide eyes took it all in.

The apparent question is: What must that have been like for her? The obvious answer is: It was too much. Lily couldn't stand still, couldn't take in any single image. Instead, she romped through the house, looking for the desired room she'd been hearing so much about: the office that, specifically for this visit, Peg had converted into a playroom. The room contained Diana's old collection of *Archie* comics; it contained her Nancy Drew paperbacks. Lily ran into that room, jumped up and down on the rubber play mat, dove into the chest of toys, squealed.

I shook off my daze, was about to order Lily to take it down a notch.

"We don't need to run." Peg already was in the hallway, her voice full of patience. "You have a whole month to play with everything. If you are calm, we can get to it all."

Lily lowered her head, wrapped her arms around her grandma's leg. Peg hugged her back, called Lily her love bug, and, with Lily still enveloping her, carried Lily's suitcase into the master bedroom, and showed Lily the special bottom drawer, cleared out just for her. Like conspiring girlfriends, they giggled about how cozy it would be, sleeping in the same bed. ("Two bugs in a rug," Lily repeated.) Lily helped Peg set the table for dinner. After dinner she followed directions and cleared the table.

RESTAURANTS WITH HIDDEN entrances and low lighting and tables that did not include squirt bottles of ketchup. Walks over the High Line, immediately followed by a few afternoon delights inside that wonderfully filthy hourly motel. Movie nights at that historic, newly remodeled theater in the Lower East Side, where Whichever Letter and I ordered curated yummies from plush seats, then, in the darkness, fondled one another. Renegade walks with the oversized pug. Sudden mad excursions to Queens. Drop-ins during the wee small hours after some press engagement had run long. Quiet decadent lingering on the couch; flirting emails that had sly memes attached to them, but also sometimes got deep; emojis both euphoric and perverse; being on the phone with one and getting a call from the other and nearly shitting myself; telling slightly varied versions of the same story in consecutive conversations; changing plans, both on the fly and out of necessity. What amounted to middling amounts of duplicity, all done to make sure that neither of these wondrous women found out about the other. God, the balancing act. The rush.

Could anyone—any fair judge—blame me? A single man blowing off some steam, while fleeing his grief, and making up for his extended, indentured servitude? It wasn't like I had a game plan, or knew what I was doing. What I had was a bunch of simultaneous ideas. Hand one: a month without Lily; of course I was eager to romp around the lush fields of Manhattan. Another part of me figured: construct a protective bubble around myself, type like hell, once in a while leave the bubble for air. Time would make things more clear, in the larger sense of what I did or did not want with each woman, what they wanted or could not handle from me. Really, that had been all I understood: writing would allow me to live, living would allow me to write, we'd see from there.

Who would have guessed: bouncing around the city on the pogo stick of my cock left my body perpetually half drained, but also had my mind continually racing and lucid. I rescheduled hanging out with my sister and her new baby multiple times; I whiffed on an appointment with a fancy foreign editor because I fell asleep upright on the couch after being up for two days straight, engaged in this twenty-four seven steel-cage death match: abandon versus introspection, adrenaline against enervation.

A's legs were tangled in my threadbare sheets. She was sitting up, leaning back against the headboard, her attention occupied by the laptop on her knees, the series of questions she had to answer, in her client's voice, for an email interview. She was munching on crackers, and was topless, and every time I looked over at her, I could not help but stare at her areola closest to me, just there, plain and everyday. I glanced away, returning my attention to the lowest bureau drawer, the long-ignored task: stuffing clothes Lily had outgrown into a trash bag. But staring at a onesie also was too much: I couldn't let myself be blinded by memories, the cuteness, how recently I'd purchased this now-obsolete little jumper.

I glanced back at A, then away from her, and explained that one of Diana's final wishes was for Lily to know her mother's side of the family.

This segued into how well Peg dealt with Lily's tantrums and, by contrast, how impossible it was to get the kid to listen to me.

"Doesn't sound *so* unique," A said, editing her email. "I mean, isn't it that way with all kids?"

Her eyes rose from the screen, caught me in full ogle. She gave that goofy smile. All I wanted to do with my life was keep that look on her face.

Only now here was Z. Bringing over a big gray pot. Standing in the kitchenette over my ancient stove, chopping celery, boiling water.

My summer cold was beyond gross, my nose stuffed through the back of my ears, wadded tissues all over the couch. Z swore on the first name of a deceased ancestor, this soup was the cure. A woman hadn't taken care of me like this since Diana before she got ill, before she became pregnant. I let Z fuss over me, listened as she related my frustration with Lily's tantrums to tantrums from her own childhood, which she then connected with disagreements she'd had with her parents while growing up. Z gave examples, shared ideas. She was in her mid-thirties. During cynical moments, I thought she might have looked at this widower dad as a long-sought answer, a no-assembly-required domestic partner. Did I mind?

She winked, played up the curative powers of her soup. "Only one part of my domestic capabilities."

AT SEVEN O'CLOCK, whatever else was going on, I made damn sure to be home, at my desk, smack in front of my laptop, for when that pair of dings sounded—first the high note, then the second one, sliding in lower, and then that familiar, oblong rectangle, expanding through the center of my screen.

Coming into pixelated focus from the desktop camera on Grandma's terminal, the shot zoomed down, capturing hair that was beyond combed, beyond neat: I could actually see a part down the middle, Lily's scalp visibly carved out like a river on a relief map. A thick braid on each side, clamped by colored ribbon, led into ponytails. Last night there had been a bun, held together with rubber bands and animal berets. How was Peg able to get her to sit still?"

"*My girl, my girl,*" I sang, the opening lyric from the closing song of Nirvana's legendary acoustic set, one of the last shows Kurt Cobain had played. Continuing to entertain myself, I added my own lyrics, shoehorning them to fit inside the line: "*Lilisita Mon Amita.*"

Her forehead, a field of pale white skin, took up a good third of the screen. She glanced up from her comic book, caught sight of me, flashed a grin, sort of. She shook out a hello wave, then went back to examining the colorful images.

"Hey there, Daddy," said the middle of Peg's torso, visible from behind Lily's chair.

The screen froze, parts of its image glitching: the straps of Lily's new dress, their little white circle patterned on red fabric. Yesterday her dress had been light blue with yellow gingham.

"Can you still hear us? Is this working? Daddy misses you. Do you miss Daddy?"

"Yes," she said.

"What did you do today?" I asked.

"Hello?" I followed up.

Swimming class at the Y; a visit to the Memphis children's museum, where FedEx had donated a *plane* for kids to run around inside. Lily's sentences were relaxed; they flowed, wound, swirled, showing her developing personality, a mind capable of imagination, making connections, working through an idea: "We are going tah visit Miss Martha tomorrow. She's doing ah singing concert. I lahkes singing, but am a dancer; I dance like Liesl. You're not supposed to run around in the rain but in *Sound of Music*, Leisl *dance*s around in the rain. Liesl is *seventeen*."

"Hold up. Am I hearing a drawl?"

Lily's eyes darted, mischievous and caught.

"You're developing a drawl?"

She giggled, then disappeared below the table.

When we reached this point, any question received the same answer. I plunged ahead anyway: "What are you guys having for dinner?"

"Good" came from beneath the empty chair.

TEN THIRTY AT night, whatever, whenever in the morning; either way, I was taking up as much space in bed as I wanted, my notepads spread out within arm's reach, my glasses—where the fuck were they? okay—atop a near pillow, me not even worrying that a temple would end up chewed, mangled, the temple separated from the frame and thrown to the floor, yet another pair of glasses destroyed. I was free to watch any stupid, vulgar thing on my laptop. Was I eating a Reese's Big Cup? Who can say?

All of a sudden deciding and heading out in the dead of night, aimless, wandering, sipping Coke straight from the can and feeling the summer breeze in my face and the humidity on the back of my neck, having the street life all around me, people buzzing, laughing, talking shit, everywhere flirting and strutting, bar-hopping techie hipsters, would-be punks hunting the latest three-star restaurants, stock market bros on the prowl for real estate, social media influencers taking sidewalk selfies, entitled New York University transplants holding court about how this city should work, and me, in the middle of it, at least partially, sort of, but also half-awash in memories: Diana and I coming down here, getting Belgian frites or eating at the communal table of that vegetarian kitchen. Oftentimes we used to remark about some beautiful couple, how it was their turn to have these streets, and how that was okay. It *had been* okay, too, then. But now, as I walked through the East Village, I'd be fully aware, in my reflection, in storefront windows: my receding hair, my sunken eyes, my aged bones. I was obviously so much older, *generations* older, foreign; indeed, for what felt like the first time, this new iteration of inhabitant felt distant to me. I'd wonder how various youngies I passed would fare if they took my class, what sort of grades they'd earn. I'd find myself drawn instead to the mother out so late with that stroller, that smart, not-young woman walking hand in hand with her aged father, the mom losing her shit at her child, himself having a tantrum in the street. I'd want to say *something*, maybe pound my heart at them, flash a peace sign, because this was it, this was how the river flowed.

Then also able to just sit at my desk, strap in, and see what kind of chaos emerged. Able to listen to the Mets on my old transistor radio with the broken antenna.

Any mother of small children who writes learns guerrilla warfare; they have to. Dads, no: Philip Roth wasn't about to lose a minute at the desk taking care of Little Bubbie. But it's not like Mom's creative life shuts down once the little wonder wakes from a nap, gets home from day care, starts demanding snacks, spreading their toys, dominating all attention through all spaces. Mommy writers have long compensated, sharing their cheat codes: how they recognize opportunities, grab scraps of time. I did not read mommy blogs because of some stupid principle (I know, I know), meaning this was one more area where I'd had to learn the hard way, what amounted to a series of DIY tactics. I'd be lying if I said they didn't have an appeal, my own curated set of tricks—like taking notes in the minutes before falling asleep, then typing them into the computer as soon as I sat down, so as to leap back into my thought process, then learning to write just keywords instead of full notes; this way I had to reconstruct the note while at the computer and, in those reconstructions, connected even more fully with my thinking . . .

Nowadays, just peck it into your notes function. Back then, my phone didn't have *apps*.

Still, this battlefield, this catch-as-catch-can mindset—the maternal, all-hands-on-deck survivalism that I'd been acclimating myself to, that I'd been living inside of ever since Diana got sick—was diametrically on the other side of the continuum from the situation

I faced now: the silence of an apartment when the child was away with Grandma, the silence that took over after I'd finished entering those notes into my computer, plus constructed new sentences to go with them, and gone and fortified those old paragraphs with new edits, and then reached that perfect situation I could move forward from, except where to, what direction?

Or the silence of an apartment after eating dinner and doing the dishes and showering and nobody else was home and the laptop screen was opened and waiting, waiting.

The silence when I'd dived down too goddamn many YouTube black holes and was hateful toward myself and no way was I going to be tempted by another one.

Lying on the couch and shutting my eyes and telling myself, *Five more minutes . . . Three more minutes . . . Ten more minutes . . .*

What it was, once again, to live inside so much stillness. To learn once again to reconnect, to look at a photo on our wall and soak in memories of Diana, those hard memories that used to make me just want to curl up in a ball and weep, and instead to take those memories and sit with them and think about their details, what I might be able to glean, repurpose, employ. Now I had the distance that was necessary for such a task. I had this silence to move through. During this uninterrupted stretch of time and space, I was learning, once again, inch by inch, how to chase, home in on, capture, the difference between a word and the right word, what Mark Twain called the difference between a lightning bug and lightning.

I opened the fridge. My eyes came upon a pouch—the same brand of organic yogurt pouch that park mothers discussed, and that I took pleasure in ridiculing. Half plastered to the top of the vegetable crisper, held in place by some sort of coalesced substance, its plastic shouted for attention, bright colors sky blue and orange.

How long had it been there? Since the spring, I guessed—when a best friend had brought yogurt pouches to the playground and Lily had started demanding her own.

Just what would it be like to live in a world where my refrigerator was free of yogurt pouches?

"IF IT'S REFRIGERATED and still before the expiration date," Crystal said, "you just wash off the goo. No biggie."

"Right," I said. "Thank you."

"I don't understand." My sister took a break from folding her laundry. "You don't have to get rid of it."

"Crystal, don't you ever just . . . not want to deal?"

My sister's bob looked a bit ratty, her blond streaks faded, her roots showing. Her bloodshot eyes had rings under them. She likely hadn't showered in a week. But her new baby had done us a solid, consenting to nap right before my visit. And her three-year-old, Declain, was in another room, occupied with his iPad. Her husband—who weeks ago had finished as an understudy on Broadway (the actor in the part had promised, "You will never get onstage")—was off at another audition; soon he'd come home and change for tonight's bartending shift. Still, though their apartment may have been momentarily calm, Crystal's exhaustion, the fullness of her overload, was apparent in how she processed my question.

"What exactly are you talking about, Charlie?"

Her oldest nickname for me, recognition that something was up.

"Maybe I'm not the person to do this," I began. "I've been thinking: What about Peg?"

The energy in the room turned, going stale. I pretended not to notice, forged onward: "First thing, seventy-plus years old, she's living on a fixed income, so it would be a big matzo ball for her. But say I got her access to Lily's monthly Social Security money. Maybe that would help with some costs. Dollars spent in Memphis have to stretch farther, yes?"

Crystal fixed her glare. Over the years, the narrowing of her eyes onto my personage had conveyed more messages than I could count. Its current meaning was unavoidable. I lowered my voice, not wanting to wake her baby over in the next room.

"And Peg has a brother; him, his wife, the extended Taylor family, they're all down in Memphis," I said, kicking into gear. "And Southern church culture. That's its own universe: there'd be youth groups, day care, all sorts of other toddlers for Lily to make friends with."

She took all this in, face frozen. "Uh-huh."

"Peggy's a member of *two* churches; that means *two* new support systems, *two* versions of a loving God to embrace Lily. All the women Peg honks at and does YMCA aerobics with, they'll definitely get involved. An *armada* of well-meaning elderly Southern church folk, all fawning over Lily, teaching her how to act, *how to be.*"

"And you've brought this up to Peg?"

I could not meet Crystal's eyes, used the opportunity to fold the sleeves on a sweater, place them atop a pile of folded clothes on her kitchen table.

"Charlie." A slight shake of her head. "You're serious?"

I kept avoiding, checked my phone—registering that three new texts awaited. I picked up the clothes pile, started toward Crystal's bedroom.

"I'm still trying to decide," I admitted. "I know she'd get a calmer life, soak in family, stories about her mom. Hell, she's already getting a Southern accent."

"You're her father."

"Peg nourishes Lily's instincts for kindness. She brings out Lily's gentle nature. I don't know that I'm doing that."

"How long are you talking about?"

"Maybe try a few months? If it works, who knows? Long weekends and holidays I could fly down."

"I guess." Crystal sipped from her diet soda. "Right now you definitely seem to have other priorities."

"Hey."

"I saw you checking your phone. And you've bumped hanging out with me *multiple* times. Where there's smoke . . ."

She took another sip, one I felt showed a decent amount of satisfaction with herself. When ready, she said, "This is not what you planned. We all know it."

"It's not like I haven't devoted every minute to that kid."

"You've been doing everything you can, Charlie. It's hard. Even with a partner. Believe me, I know. And after what you've been through—"

"I've been fucking doing it, haven't I? And how's that been working out?"

"Actually, I've been thinking about that."

Now it was my turn to stare.

"Maybe there's a connection," she said. "There's something unsettled in you. I don't know what, exactly. But when this unsettled thing radiates, it affects what happens, how things go."

"Crystal, what—"

"You love her; we all know that, Charlie. It's not like you want Lily hurt."

"What are you saying?"

"You shouldn't be parenting by yourself. Everyone sees that. No one should, but definitely not you. Still, you *are* parenting by yourself.

And you have to figure out how to accept this, you have to decide. Do you want her around? If you really don't—honestly, Charlie, is that what you're saying here?"

We were near her bedroom door now, both of us carrying stacks of folded clothes. My sister stopped. She was balancing her laundry on her arms, but she still managed to grab my wrist. Through the entirety of my adult life, Crystal had been my best friend, the person who I knew was looking out for me; more than that, among those I trusted to deliver, straight, whatever had to be said, she was first among equals.

One side of her mouth twisted. Her voice was low but strong. "I'm telling you something. Bring this up to Peg, give that woman a chance to raise Lily—even for how long?—you don't know what you're letting out of the box."

She thought about it, squinted, fixed me with her look. "This is really what you want?"

THAT NIGHT WAS night seventeen without her: yes, turns out I was counting. She wore yet another new dress, again purchased by Grandma and appropriate for one more afternoon at church. Hair up, or in braids, but as near to perfection as was possible, barely a thin strand visibly out of place on my screen. Lily told me about her day at the library. She ran out of the shot and came back with a library book, then ran away again, returning this time with a new dolly. Lily shared the dolly's name with me, and that the dolly was acting up, needed a time-out. Lily laughed at whatever I said in response; she batted her eyes, flirted, got distracted, wound down, ran out of things to say, and lingered in front of the desktop anyway, giving a crooked, almost sly smile, staring at me, wanting to stay on Skype, to keep our connection.

My stomach was a knotted metropolitan freeway at rush hour. It would have made sense to tell her it looked like she was having fun with Grandma. To ask if she felt like staying longer. I could have asked to talk to Grandma privately. *Go and do it, fool.*

"Do you want to hear about Daisy?"

She clapped. *"Daisy!"*

A new member of our world: the little witch who wanted to be good. "A student at the School for Young Witches in Wichita, Kansas," I began, starting off the riff that always began these stories. "Daisy wanted to wear a sparkly tiara instead of a pointy hat."

"And a magic wand instead of a broom," Lily said.

I had plans in Brooklyn; if I left right at that moment, I'd still end up being late.

I stayed on, told the story.

Day eighteen without her, middle of the afternoon. Instead of working through a troubling chapter in my novel, I found myself in aisle five of Kmart, a store whose presence in the East Village made me aghast, and what I was doing there was this: I was shopping for a child's desk to put in our bedroom, double-checking the measurements on the box against whatever I'd scribbled on the back of an envelope.

I imaged Lily meeting Z, how my child would take to Z's long, princessy lashes and thick curls, her pulsing, obvious charisma, to say nothing of that braying laugh. I found myself hoping—maybe half hoping—that Z and I ended up in a relationship, that Lily and Z would meet, hit it off.

Z and I joked around on the couch. She grabbed the back of my head, shoved it into her sweaty armpit. I gagged, laughed, worried: *Dear God, am I in love with her?*

Afterward we lay in one another's arms. Z started telling me about something that took place on a shoot. She unpacked another weird detail, followed by what sounded like a horrible decision. The more she talked, the more the oddness escalated; instead of a weird, funny anecdote, the story turned into a professional disagreement, one where she knew what she was doing but kept exacerbating the situation, which made no sense.

"I know you've worked with this magazine awhile," I said. "You're comfortable with these people. But you rely on them for a decent chunk of your assignments? So then—"

She looked at me like I had dirty underwear over my face. "You're on their side?"

Then it was A and a meandering afternoon. We wandered around a park in Queens, wrapping ourselves in minutiae: a certain comedian's rise through the world of alternative comedy; the different things I could do to my diet that might reduce my sodium count; exercises that might allow me to feel more healthy in my body and maybe deal with stress better. A let down her guard some, sharing the practical challenges of public relations when you were in green rooms with men who were in some stage of inebriation and felt their oats and kept coming up with the original idea to paw your ass. "I've set up a few exploratory interviews at talent agencies," she admitted. "I was thinking, maybe getting into artist management."

"You're going be an agent?"

She shrugged. She didn't really know what was happening.

"That seems to be going around," she said.

The next day we were on our laptops. Almost daring each other, we compared deals on travel websites, various hotel and airfare packages. A quick Marfa getaway? Didn't three days on a Mexican beach sound great?

"Going away together would be a concrete step forward" is what Dr. Mark Roberts said, when he heard my recount. "Is this really a serious consideration?"

I leaned backward; the leather of his couch exhaled for me, making a pained squeak.

THE SHADOW OF the Washington Square arch didn't stretch long enough to reach us, and though the park had as much tree coverage as anywhere in the city, still, the bench Kashmir and I found was open for a reason—at this hour of the day, this section of the park meant no protection. A tepid, sticky afternoon; while we had seats, the crowns of both of our skulls—middle-aged, thinning—were perspiring. We kept on crunching the dried plantains Kashmir had brought with him, watching as a trio of beautiful freaks pranced past. Neither of us allowed our necks to turn and follow.

I'd known Kashmir since grad school, more than fifteen years now, dating back to when friends called me *Chuck*. We were both young and single and used to stay up late in our dorm's communal living room, Kashmir pounding out smooth little beats on the skins while we downed cheap beer and talked shit—about literature, writers we loved, the books we'd write. Kashmir was married now, the father of two, and even in July was schlepping back and forth from Brooklyn, through Manhattan, and into New Jersey, where he taught summer session at the same private school for boys where, during the school year, he taught English. During his commute each day, he wrote and edited his novel in progress, making the changes on his phone.

Today he'd hop on the train and teach right after our meeting. "It sucks, but what can you do?" he said. "The mortgage has to be paid. You want to write, you have to figure it out."

"Gore Vidal used to tell writers who asked him about writer's block, 'Fuck off. Plenty more where you came from,'" I said. "When I was writing my first book, I used to remind myself of that all the time."

Kashmir shielded his face from the sun's heat, seemed to consider this. He reported that things were basically good. Some problems with the plotting, but he remained confident. He'd find his way through if he could just find the time to fix this draft. "My real problem, Chuck. If I just had a moment's peace. Every day when I arrive home, I swear, before the front door is shut, my wife jams her boot straight up my ass."

I munched, swallowed, listened.

"The one thing that keeps me coming home is the girls," Kashmir said, referring to his daughters. His tone changed. "They're my best friends; they keep me alive. You know how that is."

It was the ideal moment. Bring up my dilemma with Lily. Tell him about Memphis, Peg, Lily, everything.

"Can I have more plantains?" I asked.

He acquiesced, shaking more chips into my hands.

"I didn't mean to get myself in this situation," I started unloading. "Not with Lily. Not either of these women. I never expected anything so complicated. Not any of it. And I have no clue how long I can keep up this pace . . . but I'm not exactly looking to extricate myself either."

"What you are describing, two goddesses, all men our age dream about."

"Because we're too old," I said. "Isn't there something pathetic about being forty-four, chasing pussy across the city?"

Kashmir gave a thoughtful chew, the tendons in his jaw flexing. "Middle-aged men are teenagers. We see signs of our mortality, immediately old issues return, only they are stronger and we are weaker against them."

From near the fountain at the middle of the park, a flock of applause rose, apparently prompted by a street performer. We both went silent, listening. The clapping diffused; to me the sound felt like an appropriate response to Kashmir's insight. Kashmir gave a slight, comic wave, as if acknowledging the praise. Meanwhile, something else occurred: his remark dislodging a memory inside of me, one I hadn't thought of in how long.

"When I was sixteen?" I said. "There's no way to measure how much time I spent imagining. *What does it feel like to have someone's tongue in my mouth?* Sixteen years old, I didn't understand how people knew what to do, when it was okay to shove your tongue in someone else's mouth."

Kashmir's eyes flashed delight. He revealed excellent canines, a winning smile.

"These days, almost every day, I can't help but wonder: How long can I draw this out?" I paused, gathering my thoughts. "It's almost clinical. How often will I be able to see each of them? When do I need to ease off the gas? How involved do I want to get? I tell myself, *Nothing's serious.* Five seconds later: *Maybe I want to make this legit. Do I really see things getting exclusive?*"

"And what's your answer?"

"I guess the calculations fluctuate. They recalibrate—like when I left my phone in a cab, then got an excess of shit about the pictures that might be in there, if the cabbie revived my cheap dead phone and magically unlocked my password."

Kashmir drummed his knee. "Fucking hell, you left naked photos in a cab?"

"Oh, there's more," I said, then explained just what "more" meant.

"Both goddesses?" He kept staring at me. "A single day?"

"Didn't bathe afterwards. Just to keep the smell lingering."

Kashmir pursed his lips, nodded. A gaggle of healthy-looking undergraduates passed us, and we both worked hard not to look directly into their luminescence. Both of us went silent so they would not hear any of this. Kashmir poured me more chips. He clamped a hand onto my shoulder, giving it a squeeze, and I winced at his strength, remembered how he used to pound those drum skins.

"My brother," he said, "you are in the fun part of the romantic comedy. Right before the hero gets discovered. Before everything turns to shit."

IMAGINE AN OLD stone retaining wall. It threatens collapse: at any moment the landscape of its English countryside garden might tumble recklessly down into the street. That is what awaited me, at the precipice, when I opened the door of the fridge.

In the front was a cardboard pint with the dregs of an order of penne from that excellent place across the street (not much vodka sauce left, but if I nuked it long enough, it might get soft and good). Next to that, a rectangular Chinese takeout thing with condensation all over the inside of the plastic lid and a few burnt orange globules underneath, looking maybe like an unmotivated teen's obligatory science fair experiment. (Hypothesis: What happens to sweet-and-sour shrimp if you let them alone forever?) Farther to the side: baby carrots with freezer burn where the bag had been ripped open; unopened broccoli florets that were not yet all brown; bushels of organic celery (Mötley Crüe drummer Tommy Lee swears that celery kept his erections potent); a quart of green drink; a bottle of Caesar dressing with the cap off; a ketchup bottle new enough to not have gotten gunky at the top—

Did the fridge smell funky? Had I grown inured to the stench of my fridge?

I reached above and beyond that protective front wall, fumbling around until I found, half wrapped in a paper towel, a bunch of turkey burgers that I'd left on the burner for too long but could eat,

I guessed, if nothing else called my name. Then the remains of a rotisserie chicken with aluminum foil hanging off it like some sort of negligee. I found a forgotten, sealed, empty tub of cream cheese; I found unopened hummus, an opened container of guac that had the color of a small, old family pet in desperate need of antibiotics. Two bagels in a plastic bag that looked fine but probably I should devour soon. What was Smartfood popcorn doing in there? A hint of an egg carton in the back. The Brita good and full.

The bottom level wasn't quite as cluttered, but still provided more than enough reason to clean the fridge, or just grab something and shut the door and get back to my desk.

That pouch should have been easy to ignore.

Just what would it feel like to open the fridge and not see, in the bottom of my sightline, that flash of bright color?

To know exactly what I'd done—why the yogurt pouches were gone?

FOUR WEEKS AND a day after I'd taken Lily to Memphis, beneath the scaffolding on West Twenty-Third, there she was. Rushing toward me. Fake fur vest. Skirt made to look like rose petals. Knee-high socks in thick stripes, orange and pink.

Give her up and in the middle of an afternoon's procrastination, I'd know that I relinquished my daughter so I could watch a cat play a keyboard on YouTube. Chasing down a cater-waiter at some literary function, I'd know that I surrendered my kid for a bunch of small talk and a shitty-ass meatball. Posturing on some awards podium, I'd be the guy who paid for his writing life by giving away his little girl.

I lifted Lily toward my face. Joy lit up her eyes. She leaned in, touched my nose with hers, squealed, "*Eskimo kisses!*"

A thousand balloons rose to the heavens. A million doves escorted their path. My refrigerator was already a sty. Who in their right mind wants a refrigerator without yogurt pouches?

Out of the sweltering August heat. She held my hand. We led Peg into the Chelsea branch of Doughnut Plant. "This was one of Diana's favorite places to get a treat," I explained.

"It sounds wonderful," Peg answered.

Her eyes were dull, missing their normal luster. She was perspiring around the lips. Peg never moved easily, today she shuffled along. We got her to a seat. I went up and ordered Lily the same kind of donut—Tres Leches—that her mother had loved.

Lily drank chocolate milk and remarked about which of the ceramic donuts on the wall she liked the most. Peg rehydrated with a glass of water. She mentioned a landmark donut shop back home in Memphis. Her voice was both chipper and shaky; she leaned back in her seat. For a moment her stare went vacant. The cliché holds that it's easy for grandparents and sitters to be joyful with a small child because they know the visit will end. Here was the evidence, the effect of a month spent trying to keep up with a certain Tomato Tornado.

And it was while I was taking Peg in, reader, that a very odd thing happened.

Almost as if on cue, those candy-colored plaster donuts—on the wall above and behind her . . . how to put this: those donuts started *twitching*. Like, back and forth, *syncopating*.

Now their little donut hole centers puckered; they all started, uh, *humming*.

Immediately, the tourist couple at the next table jerked to their feet. In perfect coordination, the pair of tourists veered toward one another, clasping hands, looking straight ahead. The girl gave a high kick, showing off the best, most well-defined leg musculature on the planet. The couple pivoted toward our table, toward an astonished me, an overjoyed Lily.

I wasn't tripping on acid. This was happening.

Every single person in the Doughnut Plant was looking toward our table, expressing, in song and dance, the satisfaction—*the validation*—I felt at seeing Lily's worn-out grandmother. Was this a hallucination? One of those revelations that true believers are always sharing on street corners? The song's first lyric concerned all the times this child had spent me to the marrow. Dancers motioned toward precious, deflated Peg. They chanted the chorus:

> See?
> It's not just me.
> I mean, yes, it's me.
> But not just me.
> Toil for glee
> Your soul is the fee
> This shit's way hard
> It's not just me.
> Don't you *see-eee-eeeee?*

MUSICALS ARE LOVE, I've been told. Musical theater wasn't close to my area of expertise, but during my childhood, when I was no older than five, my mother sang and danced me around our kitchen, butchering lyrics to shows she loved. When Crystal turned twelve, she went into Theater Kid Mode, spending afternoons with like-minded, overly emotive friends, watching videotapes from Blockbuster. Some of that rubbed off on me. I was far from an expert; even now my thoughts on musical theater are crude and reductive. Nonetheless it's apparent to me that the musical, as a device, embodies the best urges inside of each of us. Simultaneously, the musical *channels* those best urges, doing so through some of our most joyous, moving forms of self-expression—that is, using song and dance to play out versions of the drama of *what life should be*. In real life, your job is going nowhere, lovers lie and steal, the dice are loaded, dreams go down the shitter. The art of musical theater not only allows us to cope with the disappointments we know all too well; musical theater *transcends* life's disappointments, unspooling the thinnest counter-narrative, impossibly strong thread, blindingly bright colors. Town meetings break out into song and dance; mobsters brush up their Shakespeare; the flower-selling urchin twirls around with the king; the inveterate gambler bets on love with the Salvation Army spinster; the guy who's been hunted *for decades* about a loaf of bread is key to flag-waving revolution. Protests against an illegal war turn into pleas to let the sun shine in. We get graceful men lifting lovely girls in white.

"*Someone to crowd you with love*" goes that famous song from the production about not being tied down. "*Someone to force you to care.*"

That diva from that smash twentieth-century bohemian musical (which was based on that smash nineteenth-century bohemian opera)—what does she sing? "*Today 4 U / Tomorrow for me.*"

Tony and Maria, the duet of duets: "*Tonight, tonight / The world is full of light.*"

One step further—the most famous song, probably, in all musical theater: "*Tomorrow tomorrow / I love ya / Tomorrow.*"

This was the flavor of the spirit that I wanted to cultivate inside Lily. Goodness over badness. This time it would all turn out all right.

That was why we spent time every night watching those scenes, why we returned to them.

I wanted her singing and dancing in the rain. Yes. But there was more to it. I see now. I was trying to buoy my own spirits. I was playing those videos to convince *myself*.

Well, I was convinced, finally—and in the Doughnut Plant underneath the Chelsea Hotel, of all places. I was accepting her—not just because there were no other choices, but because *she* was my choice.

CHAPTER EIGHT

THREE DAYS AFTER Peg returned to Memphis, Lily threw a fit in Walgreens when I did not purchase a toaster oven like she wanted. An employee, alarmed by the horror film screams from aisle five, sprinted toward us, poised to call the cops. Lily tantrumed harder. That night she raged against dinner, procrastinated extra about brushing her teeth, squirmed against bedtime. Waking in the dead of night, she unleashed three alarms: *"My legs hurt."* I had been recalibrated for her return, prepped to be a willing, positive dad. I coolly rubbed lotion on her hamstrings. I helped her get good and comfy back under the covers. I led her through our visualization exercise where we lay on the beach and imagined our feet in the sand, the birdies in the sky, the lapping sound of the waves coming to shore. I did the deep breathing alongside her, lay motionless in bed with her in the dark.

Back when Lily was just a few weeks old, when she was occupying the role of the baby who stayed up and cried all night, at four in the morning, Diana was up with her. Fully healthy Diana. Fully exhausted. Cuddling infant Lily, she paced the apartment, singing to her, maybe breastfeeding. Loads of tension between us—side glances, uncomfortable silences, the passive-aggressive putting away of dishes. The birth had been hugely stressful and there's no way I wasn't freaked out about the kid actually having arrived, what our lives were going to be like now, all of that. I'd tag off, take my turns with the baby, but part of that was because I knew she felt I didn't want to do it, and though she was right, I wasn't going to let her know it. So while I put in my time, holding the baby on the couch during arranged late shifts, the larger truth was, Diana had been wanting to shoulder the bulk of the responsibilities herself, trying to prove to herself that she'd be a good mother, that she *was* a good mother. I'm sure Diana was super aware of the tensions between the two of us in the house as well, which couldn't have helped. Anyway, she lost it. Holding the baby and weeping, sort of raving at Lily, exhausted, end-of-the-rope venting: "*Why won't you fall asleep? You have to fall asleep!*"

This memory reminded me it was okay that it wasn't easy for me.

I ended up dozing off in the bed next to Lily, falling asleep before she did.

The fourth night of her shenanigans, my efforts were less extravagant, my patience less fortified. Day five, Dr. Melfi squeezed me in for a special noontime meeting. "It sounds like it was an intense month for Lily," she said. "She experienced so much with her grandmother in Memphis. Wherever she looked, she saw all those pictures of her mother. That's obviously significant. Lily couldn't know how to take them, what her grandmother wanted from her, if she was supposed to replace her mother. And now she also just left her grandmother, which means leaving behind all the bonds she and Grandma just strengthened. I'm sure Lily's still processing. And she was away from you for a long time. Lily is very protective. She wants to care for you. That's a lot to put on a little girl."

I'D BEEN UNDER the impression that embracing fatherhood, deciding I wanted this, would magically change the flow of our river. I should have known: searching clouds does not mean that clouds hold answers. Maybe it was possible to alter the scene in the sky a little, though, throw in a new constellation. Maybe a change would foster different energies.

A and I hadn't ended up in Puerto Rico for that weekend; some hard feelings over that remained, not exactly what you would call a burning cauldron of passion between us. Still, our attraction was consistent—and mutual. It wasn't *not* working. After some schedule negotiations, she came over for dinner.

Lily concentrated, taking her time, making sure each stroke was straight, working to make sure A's pinkie nail was completely covered with sparkly yellow polish. A considered, blew on her hand, posed a bit, mooned with genuine glee. "It's *divine*." (After Lily was asleep that night, she'd tell me it really had been fun, allowing her a brief return to the traditions of femininity that had loomed so large through her Midwestern girlhood. "A step back on a road that I rejected, just because of some catty eighth-grade bitches.")

Once Lily's nails were done, they moved on to choosing Lily's bedtime pajamas. Lily considered, then decided against a striped shirt. A's response was measured: she told Lily about working at the Gap, showed how you folded a garment. Lily enthusiastically gave it a shot with the striped shirt. A's laughter was genuine, matter-of-fact: "Please, who doesn't get sleeves wrong?"

I took her in, digesting how reassuring, how calming, A was. We all snuggled up in bed, started watching an episode of *My Little Pony*. Lily shared how much fun it would be in the morning: "I'm going to get up early, come out to say hi to you on the foldout bed." I watched A's shoulders tense. She seemed to be looking for a way out. Nonetheless she nodded along. "Explain this 'alicorn' deal to me. The unicorn has wings? So that means it flies?"

If my heart did not quite melt, my appreciation had no limits.

But I was still seeing Z. To her credit, she had her own principles and refused to visit me at night, after Lily was asleep. "Nice try there," she'd say. We made do with nooners, sometimes followed by lunch at a burger joint in Harlem. One afternoon, on a walk with her pug, she admitted she wanted to be a mother. "That's my dream. A house full of jocks, all making chaos." I froze. *The fuck I want more of them.* It wasn't a thought or a reaction, just a brick wall. In some ways, the wall allowed for clarity, as it affirmed my most selfish instincts. This was how I felt. But did I feel this way about doing more parenting? About kids with Z specifically? Was I perhaps reacting to Z's late-night phone soliloquies, when she could be charming but also might slip, venting without pause about whoever had disappointed her that day? Had mentioning her desire to be a mother been a simple attempt at sharing something important about herself, and I was overreacting, or was it a bigger signal? I couldn't figure out whether I saw a future for us, let alone whether it was okay to introduce Z to Lily—to say nothing of what might be the right way to do so.

Still, toward the end of August, I gave in. A brutally hot Sunday afternoon. Lily and I loitered outside the Disney Store in Times Square.

"When's she going to be here?" Lily asked.

Six feet away from her, on the other side of a plexiglass window, an entire galaxy of wonders awaited. Her eyes were wide. She bit her lip. Her hand was damp with sweat and held on to mine, until I let go of hers, wrote out another text.

"Just a little longer," I said.

Answers were infrequent. Then came apologies. To her credit, Lily remained the most loyal of soldiers, shifting from one little foot from another, awaiting the order to charge.

One more ping: Z and the driver could not figure out how to find the Disney Store in Times Square.

Reader, we stood on that sidewalk for well past thirty minutes. You try it. Try keeping a four-year-old—even the best of troupers—from entering the Disney store on an August afternoon for more than half an hour.

What was best for Lily? I vacillated, turned silent and inward, unable to explain to either woman that I not only was measuring her, but was contrasting her with another. With friends, though, I could be voluminous, so much so that they zoned me out, nodding weakly. *Maybe you shouldn't be with either of them* was a reply that stayed in my brain.

Thirty minutes into a late-night call, I heard A's eyes rolling. "*Sorry?* Like I haven't heard *that* before."

Lunch. Z stabbed at her tabouli. "You fade away, then reappear. Everything's supposed to be all fine."

A: "I don't doubt that you're well-meaning."

Z: "*Now* you're present. *Now* you're here."

A: "You have a lot on your plate. I get it."

Z: "Am I totally on board for those kamikaze lunch dates? Yes, I am."

A: "I think I'm understanding up the wazoo."

Z: "—and I don't have any problem scheduling around those preordained sitter nights."

A: "But when I need *you*?"

Z: "Kind of available."

A: "*Half*-available—"

Z: "You get all reluctant."

A: "You're just *trifling.*"

Z: "Which just makes no sense—"

A: "It's like we take one step forward—"

Z: "Then you scurry back into your hole."

A: "It pisses me off *so much.*"

Z: "I can't rely on you."

A: "*So* unreliable—"

Z: "I mean, it's almost like you're seeing somebody else."

A: "But there's no way. You can't be that much of a shit."

"WELL THEN, HOW much do you care for A?" Dr. Roberts wanted to know.

"I don't know how to answer. We have good times. Other times I . . ."

"Go on," he said.

"Believe me, I'm more than aware she's been thrown into the deep end. I can't tell you how thankful I am. A hangs in there, treading water—as opposed to, what, dog paddling over to the side of the pool and leaping out and running like hell?"

"Noted."

"Maybe I'm being hypersensitive. I'm just responding to my own, what, overcompensating? But the connection between her and Lily—in particular, how tense A gets. I see it. And once I see it, I can't unsee."

My therapist answered with conviction. By continuing things with A, I was making an implicit promise. The effort she was making may have been of her own free will. However, if I cared about her well-being, I had to be considerate of the emotional commitment that went into her efforts.

One way or the other, I had to be fair to her.

"Fuck me," I said.

BUT THEN Z and I were at a thing, it doesn't matter what, just that Terri Jay Cello was babysitting, and I'd given a concrete time for our return.

"What's she going to do?" Z asked. "Leave your kid home alone?"

She'd used this line more than once. It was a way of trying to extend the evening, trying to keep our thing going.

Tonight it struck me in a bad place.

Not long after Diana had passed, a posting had led me to the poet Diane di Prima's memoir, *Recollections of My Life as a Woman: The New York Years*. Di Prima tells the story of a night Allen Ginsberg was having a party: Jack Kerouac and a few other big names were in town. The evening promised to be, as di Prima put it, "one of those nights with lots of important intense talk about writing you don't remember later." She got a friend to babysit her young daughter and promised to be home by 11:30 p.m. That night turned out to be everything you'd want from a high-end literary beat party. Kerouac was half-crocked, to the point where he was stretched out on the linoleum. When the clock hit the magic point, di Prima started saying goodbye. Kerouac raised himself onto an elbow and announced, "DI PRIMA, UNLESS YOU FORGET ABOUT YOUR BABYSITTER, YOU'RE NEVER GOING TO BE A WRITER."

Horrible, right? The defining utterance of an entitled male asshole.

"I considered this carefully, then and later," di Prima wrote, "and allowed that at least part of me thought he was right. But nevertheless I got up and went home . . . I'd given my word to my friend, and I would keep it. Maybe I was never going to be a writer, but I had to risk it. That was the risk that was hidden (like a Chinese puzzle) inside the other risk of: can I be a single mom and be a poet?"

Obviously, I didn't have to choose between writing and parenting. Where di Prima was clawing to enter and exist within a foreign world, the world of male writers, during an era when male writers were, pretty much, everything, my writing may have taken a hit, sure, but while I'd been resentful, I'd also recognized there wasn't an absolute, either/or situation. No, I was trying to enter a different separate land. In its own way, this might have been an equally hostile place, seeing how a prenatal umbilical connection with my daughter was something I most def did not possess. Most of the time, I had jack squat natural instincts about what to do. I guess in this way, I can claim to have been like di Prima at that party in that I was trying hard, but firmly out of my element.

There's a good argument that when Z asked, "What's she going to do?" more than simply trying to keep our evening going, more than wanting to further our bonding, in point of fact Z was fighting for our relationship out on the sidewalk, brawling for the domestic future she wanted with me, doing so in this instance by offering me an out, appealing to that selfish me, the me that wanted to stay longer, to spend time in the world with a beautiful woman.

Was that *so* selfish?

I gave enough, didn't I?

I remember screaming at Z on the street in the middle of the night.

"Fuck over someone who does you a favor? Who are you? Fuck your friends, next time, tell me, who's going to answer the call?"

I GOT HOME late, a few minutes, nothing substantial. The bedroom door was closed, meaning Lily was asleep. The living room was equally subdued: dim lights, Terri Jay Cello on the couch, wrapped in an Indian blanket, near the rattling, blasting air conditioner. Her lower face was lit by the blue glow of her laptop.

She looked up. "Something happened."

Terri Jay got up and took two steps toward the other side of the window, the orange wooden bookcase modules. She motioned toward the middle shelf.

The red velvet box was open like a clam. Out, next to it: the vase.

"Lily asked me if I wanted to see her mommy," said Terri.

"Excuse me?" As I asked, I knew I should worry.

"I didn't realize what was happening," Terri Jay said. "I thought Lily was going to show me pictures of Diana. But she led me to the box. I started to tell her no. Then I thought about it. I took out the vase. I told her it wasn't safe for her to touch. But Lily started to get upset. She wanted to see her mommy. She said her mommy was in there."

All at once: the horror of what I was being told; the sickening sensation of being told it at the end of this of all nights; and, worst of all, the separate and very significant difference between the mother Diana would have been and the realities I was trying to force into being acceptable.

I ran my hand back over my forehead, rubbed my palms into my eyes.

"I'm sorry, Charles. I had the thought, *Why shouldn't she?*"

I was going to vomit. Any second.

"I unscrewed the lid," Terri Jay continued. "I showed her. I did. We talked to Diana. Lily said, 'Hi, Mommy.' She and I both said we missed her. Lily told her mother she loved her."

"That's intense."

She shrugged. "It just seemed"—Terri was near tears—"why say no?"

MY MIND WAS not on a razor's edge that night, but since it wasn't powering down, either, I followed its directives, and stayed up well past my self-imposed curfew, preparing for yet another awkward, loving conversation that I had to initiate. Stress my love for her, that much was clear. Encourage her to talk to the vase whenever she needed. To put her hands on the vase, if she felt that was necessary. But I also had to be clear: this vase was heavy. It was a bad idea—a very bad idea—to pick up this vase. We wanted to keep this vase here with us. We wanted Mommy all in one place.

The living room was all wall shadows and midnight hues.

I don't know when or just what possessed me, but soon I headed over to the modules, stood in front of the velvet box, and put my hands on each side of the top of the urn. It's not like I put a lot of thought into this; at the same time, I was alert to what I was doing. More than alert. It was almost as if these movements had been laid out for me, I was just following along to predetermined dance steps on the floor. However, I don't want to deny my agency: I was conscious, aware, wanting to see what would happen.

Though I'd just scribbled out notes for tomorrow's conversation, including remarks about the weight of the urn, still, when I picked up that thing, I was surprised. How heavy it was. How smooth. How well-made. I pressed on its rim, turning until I got that soft metallic release. Then I opened the lid. The edges of the plastic bag were crumpled; it took me a moment to find the opening. I placed my finger. Pressed. The ash was fine; at the same time there was a roughness to it. Softer than gravel, just as dry.

A film coated my fingerprint. I raised it toward my face.

I've never admitted this. Never talked about it with anyone. But I opened my mouth.

My wife's ashes felt chalky on my tongue. They had a bone-dry taste, one that was pointed, unpleasant. Not even distinct—not something I recognized, say. But the taste of something that did not age, that remained outside the rules of time. The ashes tasted rotten. Forbidden. The ashes in my mouth were not meant to be tasted. They were not meant to be swallowed.

LAMPPOST SHADOWS LENGTHENING across the pavement; the rim of sky darkening that much earlier; shorts and tees folded into plastic bins, stored under the bed.

"When is A going to visit again," Lily asked.

"Why isn't Z coming over anymore?" Lily wanted to know.

You tell yourself you are the good one. You are the hero of this story. Certainly, you don't think of yourself as the villain in other stories that are out there.

But those stories are being told.

A late-night phone call. "You'll never guess where I am," A said. I knew somewhere in the upper Midwest, supposedly visiting her parents. I asked if she'd been drinking. "You could say that." She revealed the answer: on her former campus, wandering the halls of her old communications department. A announced each step as if doing a play-by-play. She slurred a bit, meandering, anecdotal, wanting to stay on the phone.

Her sloppiness took me aback. I felt as if some kind of boundary had been crossed, that a familiarity was being assumed—worse, was being taken advantage of. Okay, she was having a hard time being back home, a completely reasonable reaction: Who doesn't feel it in some way or another? But her neediness put me on alert. I envisioned a door—to drunken forays? to what else?—being opened.

What I thought was: *That's enough for me.*

The afternoon Z was performative for a waiter in a manner that wasn't quite flirting, but still made no sense, a message I could not decipher.

On their own, they don't stand up. Not as reasons to end a romance.

Not unless you've been auditioning those women, constantly thinking about down the road.

Z was irate—with how things ended, and that I had ended them. "Who do you think you're pulling this on?"

By contrast, A went silent; we simply went our separate ways.

On one particular side of the road, the impact was apparent: Lily kept picking out her outfits, but didn't show the same engagement, settling quickly for the first or second thing she saw. She sat at her little table and held her crayon and sort of spaced out, occupied in her own world. Her head hung at an odd, unhappy angle. I went to sit with her, joining in her art project. Rather than encouraging me to cut along the lines, Lily got loud and bossy. She waved her arms, knocking over her full glass of water. She started having similar problems spilling drinks, dropping cups. We came up with a saying, "Two hands, no spills." Still she spilled.

I knew to give her time; she was making a big adjustment. At the same time, these adjustments were already entrenched, recurrent happenings in her life—yet another cool sitter landing that real job, no longer arriving on Wednesday nights. To Lily they hadn't been sitters, none of them; they'd been friends. And they'd all left her. More female figures who weren't part of her days anymore.

I couldn't explain to Lily why this was happening.

"I JUST—I JUST keep reminding myself of the larger question. The more important question."

Dr. Roberts took the bait: "And that is?"

"Would Diana have wanted either of these woman raising Lily?"

This was my finishing move, my conversation ender, my official way out. Only Dr. Roberts did not wait to pounce.

"Isn't that a cop-out?" he asked.

I couldn't believe what I'd heard, looked at him like he was nuts.

"You were fucking two women. Each of them was invested. Wholly. At points in their lives where this mattered."

"Well—"

"And though it's certainly your right to decide neither was the right one for you—"

"For me and *Lily*," I said.

Dr. Mark Roberts furrowed his brow. I could tell he was measuring his next step.

"Three weeks ago you were ready to let Lily stay with her grandma indefinitely."

"*Mark.*"

"Maybe there's an argument that recognizing what she means to you is a step forward for you—"

"HEY."

"Okay. Let's put aside Lily for a moment."

"Why are you going so hard on me?" I asked. "Where is this coming from?"

A few seconds straightening his tie, his actions almost acted as a resetting. "I've been listening to this for a while now. I don't have to stay neutral. You up for some tough love? Come on. It's actually kind of fun."

I studied him—him and that goading, satisfied grin.

He began: "You never revealed to A or Z that there was someone else, did you?"

My silence acknowledged this truth, yes.

"For your own growth, it's worth recognizing that whether or not you were in any kind of official or recognized relationship—and I'm talking about with either of these women—you weren't being fair. You weren't an honest actor."

"Recognized," I said.

"Any claims toward a larger decency, any moral authority, or any sort of a mature perspective, they all go out the window when you are not honest." He let that sink in, continued. "Oftentimes, not being honest comes from the impulse to not take responsibility—for your actions, for your decisions."

Making sure I was following, Dr. Roberts sort of rolled his hand, as if guiding me into his next point. "Admittedly, you've already got more responsibility with Lily than you know what to do with, which is especially hard, seeing that you're someone who's spent a considerable amount of your adult history avoiding responsibility."

"This tough love stuff's a blast," I said.

"I know it's difficult. But it seems possible to me that, deep inside, you knew you couldn't handle anything substantial. Irrespective of whatever shortcomings there might have been, you nonetheless put unreal expectations on each of these women. Whether or not they did anything to disappoint you, they were going to disappoint."

"Because when they disappoint me, I get to bail."

He nodded. "It seems quite possible to me that you haven't properly grieved losing Diana. Maybe there's no way to do that. But a healthy relationship will be impossible until you do."

Dull pain. A drilling, heading into my skull, through my cortex. Whatever I'd last eaten was not happy in my tummy. I tried to stay focused, to listen to this chattering man, all these truths I did not want to hear.

CHAPTER NINE

"Oh, there's hope, an infinite amount of hope, just not for us."

—Franz Kafka

BUT SAY YOU were an entirely different species of hardbacked insect—one being forced to face the gaping maw inside himself, a cockroach unable to process hard truths, unwilling to grow into an adult member of his species. You were a parent to boot. And as a parent, no matter how much you may have admired Mr. Kafka's oeuvre (basically the dude dramatized a psychological state, before it had been officially defined for the world), no matter how much you related to his portrayal of man's alienation from this absurd and beautiful world, you nonetheless recognized an inherent fallacy embedded into that particular joke.

When you were a parent, hope arrived every fall, announcing itself with resonant alarm bells, with flyers for back-to-school sales. Hope was the long manila envelope that I'd taken out of my desk, and was busy stuffing: with the previous month's utility bill, with copies of my lease, my late wife's death certificate, my daughter's birth certificate, with any other documents that might help establish, without doubt, that Lily would be granted a seat at the school two streets and one avenue from our apartment.

Sure, I was more than a little broken. I was hoping nonetheless.

That spring—around the time I'd started seeing A and Z—Lily
and I had actually visited Public School 40. Online websites had
awarded a gold star to the school, making note of its progressive
principal, its experienced teachers, its thriving parent-teacher asso-
ciation. The school had put on a special night devoted to incoming
kindergarteners. All the dearies were even asked to bring in their
favorite stuffed animals. Lily brought her Dorothy/Wicked Witch
combo doll. After being guided through a classroom tour, the children had been all grouped and taken off to other rooms in which
they met their eventual teachers. Parents stayed put and were given a
different orientation. I wedged myself into one of those little chairs,
looked around at the walls jammed with posters and motivational
sayings, the packed shelves, the overstuffed cubbies, the classroom
appearing to me as ancient, dusty, bedraggled, innocent, sweet, deeply
charming, thrillingly alive.

Someone had knocked on the door, peeking in. "The parent of
Lily Bock?"

Lily had become nervous during the tour and thrown up all over
her doll, all over herself. Needing to be cleaned off, crying, she'd taken
my hand: "*I want to go HOME.*"

But that had been, what, however many months ago?

Who doesn't get nervous when they really want things to go
right, when they want to show their best?

We were in autumn now, time of parental hope, everyone ready
for a new beginning: new chances, new learning, a new teacher,
new friends.

This is what I told myself.

In the ankle-length cherry blossom dress that her grandma had
purchased, Lily looked both immaculate and picturesque; I managed
her hair into a reasonable bun. The school itself took up almost an
entire block, truly looking ancient and cavernous and like a warehouse

where Dickens would stash orphans. Lily got impatient on the front steps but, then, listened to me anyway, holding still long enough for a few pictures.

In those pictures, she smiles tightly, glances to the side, holds up the little handwritten announcement, the first day of kindergarten.

Another image now, also captured on the rectangular screen of what, at the time, was a recently purchased, refurbished, unlocked iPhone:

Untold children, all between the ages of four and six, sit and stand all over a rug blocked in primary colors. In the front of the picture, seated third to the left, Lily, leaning in. New classmates tower all around her, looming over her, even the ones who are sitting. The larger ones appear to be double her size. Turns out, New York City public schools are singular in that they use New Year's as their separation point between grades. This seems a small thing until you look at this picture. Lily's December birthday has her on the wrong end of the cutoff, serving as the reason the kids in the picture are so much bigger, why she looks that out of place.

That is, except for her grin: Lily grins *so wide*, that smile does not just dominate but distorts her lower face.

Later, my first instinct was *Meh, flip ahead past this image, check out the next shot.* Only, that expression . . . how hard she was trying, her effort like so much helium inside the balloon of her face, literally inflating Lily's features, pumping them beyond the point of distortion . . .

THE FIRST FRIDAY of the month, parents were invited to come into the class for the first half hour. Once again I was back, immersed amid them: their performative kindness and blatant self-interest; their corporate wear or corporate casual; their oversized knits and yoga pants; their baseball caps and tight ponytails and designer mom jeans; their mussed, unwashed hair, thick knit scarves, sweatshirts with the profile of our first Black president. Our children's writing samples were tacked along the classroom walls, simply written numbers again and again across the line. We mingled, loitered, taking in the scrawls, pretending to care, to be impressed by each and every little Einstein. It's possible I stared a count or two too long at some of the mothers, imagining their mommy lives, the size of Mommy's apartment, what Mommy's rent was.

One was looking right at me. We almost made eye contact, only she broke away, talked in a low voice with the woman next to her, made a subtle nod—at which point something inside my gut swiveled. I imagined her saying, *That skeevy guy.* My thoughts raced: Had I talked with her before, maybe while our kids played in the park? I wasn't someone who hit on moms while our kids were playing in a park—God, I hadn't done that, had I? Maybe I'd revealed too much to her? Had I been too obviously looking to be saved? Or had I been on edge, anticipating events going wrong, making cutting remarks under my breath ("*Goddamn it, Lily, what now?*")? Maybe I'd just been minding my own beeswax, hanging around the margins of whatever museum or kid's deal it had been, alone, looking like a disturbing person, looking for kids to grab, or just looking like the exact schlub I happened to be: rumpled, uncomfortable, aging, thinking of not one but *two* women I'd just loused things up with. I was missing being touched, missing the swell of a hip. I was the shellshocked poor bastard, still trying to figure out just what had happened.

Obviously, the big question about kindergarten handwriting is: How does my kid's stack up? The answer was plain as white bread. The other writing was crooked, rudimentary, but basically straight lines. Gripping a pencil was still hard for Lily; even the plastic guard thing only helped so much. She'd put in extra time, sitting at the little table in our living room, sliver of tongue peeking out of the corner of her mouth, repeating each step of Mrs. Ambriss's instructions, making sure she started right at the bottom solid blue line.

"Who effing cares," I mumbled to the guy alongside me, who was also looking at the wall, one of maybe five fathers in the room. "Big picture, she's going to figure out how to write."

He was a decade younger than I was, dressed in Friday business casual, obviously restraining himself from checking his phone, from jumping back into whatever his business was. He answered me from the throat, an agreeable smirking sound.

LILY ADORED HER new teacher; she was enchanted by having her own cubby for her coat and lunch. She performed her class responsibilities with cardiac seriousness, even if her responsibility was nothing more than being the caboose in the class line. Still, convincing her to eat breakfast on a school day was a power struggle, getting her sweater facing the right direction a physical chore. Finding her shoes, remembering her backpack, navigating out the door, walking her the eight minutes to school so she would not be tardy—every single day, this became a combination of trench warfare and dental surgery performed on me, by my kid, while Visigoths charged our foxhole.

"Jam on it," I called.

We set out. I held her hand, setting the pace for us, busting out more lyrics from eighties hip hop. "J-j-j-jam."

Lily shuffled, slowed her gait. I slowed mine, waiting for her, turning back to her. "Today you are going to be kind," I said. "You'll be a good listener."

Lily's eyes brimmed with defeat. Her shoulders slouched.

Our Sturm und Drang continued like this, each school day, all the way onto Second Avenue, when, like clockwork, we'd approach that familiar stand. A street or two in front of the school, it blocked a decent chunk of the avenue; four months of the year, it was probably out there, whether it was to hawk apartment-ready Christmas trees, oversized Easter baskets, Fourth of July inanities, or, of course, pumpkins.

Different days, reality split off, heading in new directions:

Monday	Wednesday
Maybe half a block ahead, just on the far side of the stand, Lily saw a girl from her class. My daughter was in her yellow raincoat and cloud-printed tights, wearing rain boots at least one size too big for her (because I needed them to last another year). She yanked her hand from my grip. Elbows and knees flew, boots clomped, the same motions I'd seen her make while chasing countless children through untold playgrounds. It was the sweetest thing: the purity of her desire, the fullness of her effort, hope—for friendship.	Slowing further, stopping in place, willfully staring through other kids and parents . . .
	When I was seven, my brothers and I got caught shoplifting from a local drugstore. My dad had to leave work and pick us up. When he got us home, he took me over his knee. I'd only known my dad as genial, gentle. Certainly, I'd never known his unleashed, full-grown-man strength. When he paddled my bottom, his intensity, his *power*, was shocking—not only for the spanking's physical impact, but because he introduced me to a new understanding: a high floor to which kids were not privy, where adults made adult decisions, took adult actions. It was a stark introduction to my piddling place in our much larger universe. That afternoon, I couldn't sit.
But the other child was too far away for Lily to catch up. It was obvious to anyone—anyone but Lily. Recognizing this, something inside me wilted. I was a man forcing himself to wake from an uncomfortable dream; indeed, it was all I could do to	
	In a million years you never

shake out of it and shout, "RED LIGHT"—ensuring that Lily would stop before the curb, would not run out into traffic. could have told me I'd one day lose my shit and grab my daughter, pulling her by the wrist just to get her to school.

We were trying. We were a team. Each of us
going through this together, each of us
going through this alone.

THAT NIGHT, I cued up a clip from the seventies, Madeline Kahn and Grover, one of our favorites. The legendary actress and the puppet went back and forth, singing about echoes ("*Sing what I sing, sing after me / Be my echo if you can be*"). Along the way she was tender, so sly and self-aware at the same time, flirting with Grover, with the *Sesame Street* crew, with life itself. For the entire five minutes Kahn was luminous, the segment beyond delightful. But as we watched, I grew progressively sadder, heavier. I felt myself wavering, nearing a brink.

Was the frequency, the severity, of me losing my temper at Lily offset by the depth of our relationship?

Was there a boundary line between punishment and abuse?

Maybe my actions today just flowed along in the wash of childhood, normal small parts of a much larger story?

Or maybe they did more.

Stars glowed across the darkened ceiling. Tilted colors projected from our lopsided night-light.

I held Lily's hand long past the end of video time. Her tiny fingers were light with perspiration, her skin still infant-soft. I could feel the delicate twigs of her bones beneath. I looked away from the ceiling, stared at her moon cheeks, her face in profile.

That was what I could do. I could be present. Look at her. Hold her hand.

I could listen, and breathe, and keep listening.

"When are you going to do better?" she asked.

I tried to breathe, could not breathe.

Her eyes a placid lake, focused on me.

"After we fight, you tell me you are going to do better. When will you do better?"

I did not share that I was struggling, just like her.

I did not tell her that I hated my life.

I said, "I'm trying." I managed to share the other truth, the largest truth. "I love you more than anything."

"Nobody comes anymore."

"I know."

"It's *not fair*."

I choked up. "It's not."

Those eyes remained focused. Her lips, chapped in their thickest middle, stayed a bit apart.

"It sucks," I said, clearing my throat. "Life sucks sometimes."

I added, "You have every right to get upset."

I continued: "We also need to be thankful for the time we get with our friends."

Then I said, "Isn't it nice to know that fun people, *meaningful* people, can pop into your life? Anytime. All the time."

"Why don't I get to have a mom?"

Deep breath. Three one thousand. Two one thousand . . .

"Your mother loved you." My voice broke. I stressed these next words. "She loved you more than anything. She fought so hard to be around for you, Lily. She wanted to be your mother more than anything.

"You get to be sad," I said. "But that is not all you get to be."

WHEN LILY WAS finally asleep, I emerged into my living room, sat at my desk, and found salvation, eventually, by and large, through Facebook. I know. I know. I look back, it sounds ridiculous, feeling the desire to be more social and choosing, as an answer, Mark Zuckerberg's algorithm factory. Probably it was just as stupid at the time.

But Peg, bless her heart, had included my name in a tag, thus making sure I saw the picture, a poster that a friend had made for her daughter.

Not only did I see it. That night I used Magic Markers and red construction paper, and reprinted the thing:

HOW TO HAVE A DAY OF YESSES
Don't worry about things NOT being.
Be Polite and kind to other people
Be a good listener
Don't yell unless you or someone else is in DANGER
Don't be bossy! Work TOGETHER as a TEAM
Don't get angry when someone says NO. Find something else to do

On a sheet of yellow paper, I added:

Stay calm
Greet each challenge with a smile
Deep breaths. Breathe out. Repeat
You are a determined girl
You can do ANYTHING

The following morning. Lily came into the living room, saw the charts on the wall. "What are they?"

As soon as she heard the title of the first one, her brow furrowed. She crossed her hands over her chest.

I kept reading to her.

Lily stomped to her desk, pulled out her own sheet of construction paper, uncorked a marker, and plopped herself down on the floor.

She set to writing, tentative lines, leading to segmented, broken letters:

How to Hav e aDay
oF a Day av noes
Be me n
Trt Pbl Mnly
Kr ya lt
Do ntcay yes
Onl yn
ignre Plbpl
Do not hv Pan
BeFMr donot xoaFa Mtat
dontlK tegue stan Fr nybdy

IT WASN'T QUITE 8:00 a.m. We had a whole day ahead.

I looked at that jumble of misshapen effort and felt more delight than I had in a long time. I had the overwhelming urge to hug Lily. For whatever reason, I thought of Dr. Melfi telling me, "You can't ruin this child." Here, via Lily's shaky letters, was proof positive.

At the same time, a wind twisted through my innards. A voice answered Dr. Melfi, saying: *Just watch.*

Lily was waiting, brow scrunched, eyes boring in, challenging me to react. I knew this look all too well: it was *mine*, once again, my own defiance.

Here was another moment that could split, heading in different directions. When I responded, was I going to further alter our route or would I get us back on track?

Because maybe the poster was just the normal actions of a kid asserting her independence.

Maybe it was something deeper? An indicator of more problematic defiance?

Would letting this slide allow her to get away with behavior that, however cute, was also problematic?

Would confronting Lily cement her opposition? By overreacting, would I take us further off course?

None of these were formed thoughts, just synapses working on blast.

Jesus, I didn't want another day of war.

Time was ticking. How was I supposed to answer?

It didn't seem like things were going in the right direction—not this morning. Also in a larger sense. Things didn't seem to be going right with how Lily was progressing.

And she wasn't the only one having days of no.

I'd put on my big-boy undies and accepted the responsibility, made the conscious decision to parent her, did every possible thing I could think of, and still each day carried decent odds that I'd erupt, melt down, run off anyone who might care about us, and cap the evening with a swallow of my dead wife's ashes.

"Can I have your poster, please?" I asked.

Lily was wearing pink onesie pajamas with footsies. Her shoulders were tight and scrunched up, her arms crossed in front of her chest. She did not budge. I took in her furrowed brow, her flaring little nostrils, her chubby cheeks, the whole vision of her, defenses up, armaments ready. Reader, it got me: her difficulty, her obstinance. Impossible lightness filled my chest, my heart. Maybe this was one more observation that would have been common sense for any other parent: *difficulty is part of the charm.* But for me it was a realization, a new understanding, although yes, Lily charmed me all the time, and, certainly, me wanting to laugh at her wasn't new. What was new for me was the simultaneity: being at once awestruck *and* irritated, entertained *and* horrified, so deeply in love with this little girl, wanting to guide her, wanting to burst out laughing at her, to save her, and also wanting to run like hell in the opposite direction, the rolling stone in that Temptations song an aspirational goal for me—*wherever* I'd lay my hat would be home. Except that I needed to stand there. To watch her and let her be, to appreciate my girl, Lily, being herself, and the sweet hellish totality of what this meant.

Heading over, I gently reached for the paper.

"Please?" I said.

Her grip was rigid. "HEY."

I did not pull hard, got the poster free.

Still no singing donuts. This wasn't some charming musical sequence. Just her repeating, "*HEY.*"

Two steps to get back over to the wall. I felt numb; at the same time, I felt myself plummeting.

Where were we headed? Was this all veering out of control? Maybe so. Don't the best love stories perpetually straddle that edge?

I withdrew pushpins from some other wall drawings.

"Yeses and noes," I said. "Side by side. Each one alone. Both in this together."

On the wall of our living room, I pinned this new, tender page.

CHAPTER TEN

OCTOBER 12, 1962. One week after leaving her husband and moving with her children to London, Sylvia Plath, age thirty, wrote a poem in longhand about her father, Otto Plath. (He'd passed when Sylvia was eight.) Plath compared her dead father to items including a black shoe, a bag full of God, a vampire, a Nazi, and a swastika; she labeled herself a Jew going to Auschwitz, titled this poem, "Daddy." For a decent chunk of her adulthood, Sylvia had been diagnosed as clinically depressed. She'd been institutionalized, had received electroshock therapy. In the poem she explicitly connected Otto to her former husband, and flat out blamed her father for her unhappy marriage. The narrator of the poem had to be rid of both men, had to kill both father and husband: "If I've killed one man, I've killed two——" "Daddy" ends with a stake in Daddy's "fat black heart": "Daddy, Daddy, you bastard, I'm through."

Four months after writing the poem, Plath put her head in an oven and ended her own life. Both of her children were home.

"Daddy" has long been a lodestar for gifted girls with propensities for melodrama, an inspiration for emotionally scarred young women with a desire to express their pain through art. Really, it is a touchstone for anyone, particularly young females, with an axe to grind at their family patriarch—as well as the patriarchy in general.

All of which is valid. No one claims otherwise.

If you are a father, though, this poem is an absolute terror.

It is the written embodiment of everything you do not want your grown daughter thinking about you. Simultaneously, the events surrounding the poem's writing act as an embodiment of what you do not want happening to your grown daughter. The total, worst-case scenario: what might happen if you are too strict, if you do not listen to your child, if you are absent—even if you are present in your daughter's life but cannot have a relationship with her as a young adult or as a mature adult because you die too soon. (Doctors in Plath's time didn't know how to treat diabetes properly, plus along the way you might have gotten gangrene and had to have your leg chopped off—all of which happened to Plath's dad, who, though German and strict, was not an actual Nazi.)

You do not want your little girl putting her head in the goddamn oven.

You don't want her life ruined, period, and you sure don't want her looking for reasons why.

And, okay, you know you are going to fuck it up some—like that Larkin poem promises: "They may not mean to, but they do." But you surely don't want your daughter ascribing her fucked-up marriage, let alone her fucked-up life, to actions you took, for instance, in the middle of an emergency when she was four and you were freaked and trying to protect her.

"Daddy" is near the farthest end of the toxic masculinity continuum, next to the locked-in-closet nightmares, the leather belt spankings, the molesters.

The other side, however, represents a kid left on her own.

No guidance. No assuring hand to help her.

OCTOBER 19, 2012. A week or so before Halloween, the wind picked up, as did news reports: a tropical storm was becoming more intense, approaching the Eastern Seaboard. This wouldn't be good. Broadcasters listed steps to make sure your family was safe. In our home, however, the pressing question was: Would we still get to go to the West Village on Sunday? Sunday was the day of the annual Halloween festival there, the posh boutiques up and down Bleecker Street opening their gilded doors, distributing candy to the costumed offspring of entitlement. A woman who did wardrobes for movies lived in our building; she went out of her way, procuring for Lily a Disney Cinderella dress, truly to die for, shimmering metallic blue, replete with frilly shoulders and hip flounces. I went on eBay and scoured up a tiara of plastic jewels, some silky elbow-length gloves, also light blue paper booties that covered her sneakers. Staring at her reflection in the mirror, Lily beamed ten thousand watts.

During the bus ride across town to my sister's place, she told me, "I don't like peanuts so you can have all my Snickers." I sort of mumbled approval—it was the third time she'd said this—and kept gazing out the window: the overcast sky, the western rim of Union Square, trees appearing as dark shadows, their bare branches swaying in the wind.

We made sure the kids didn't grab too many candies, thanked all the shopkeepers—those quick, perfunctory thank-yous even as their little bodies were starting for the next shop. Lily and Declain booked ahead; Crystal and I called out, reminding, "We have to be able to see you."

At the park, the festival was going full blast, running kids and stray costume parts anywhere you looked. Lily got her face painted to look like a kitten. She waited to get her hair done in the French braids I had neither the patience nor dexterity to manage. We all took a hayride around the block.

The next evening, with alerts about the storm all over the web,

I made a final run on the local drugstore for extra batteries. At the bodega, we got extra bags of Pirate's Booty, boxes of mac and cheese, anything edible still on the shelves that wouldn't need refrigerating (in the event power stayed out awhile). Afterwards, I fastened Lily inside our trusty if beaten-up stroller; we set off for an Italian restaurant in the Flatiron District. I'd become friendly with the agent of a writer I worshipped; the agent was in town to sell books to editors. Another friend, Amber, would join us. (Whenever she visited, Lily referred to her as "Glamber.")

Rain hadn't started falling when Lily and I got to the restaurant, but the staff was boarding up the front windows, removing tables from the back patio. The place was open, and if all the tables were nearly empty, they were still covered in white tablecloths. The restaurant had a full freezer of meat, fresh pasta, vegetables. "Take your time," the waiter said, lighting the candles at our centerpiece. "Work has to get done, with or without you." Rather than let food spoil, they kept hauling out loaded plates, extras gifted on top of our ordered meals, even as staff bustled to lock the place down. A waiter brought crayons; Lily colored, stopped, picked up again, returned her attention to the agent and Glamber, trying to follow, even sliding into their conversation: "I hope the storm isn't too bad. We got groceries for if it is. I bring my coins from Change Lake to the store. I get a chocolate ball but today my friend gave me it, so I did not have to pay."

Lily leaned toward the various complex dishes, sniffed, scrunched her brow, crinkled her nose. She asked what each person was eating. No, thank you, she did not want to try. Shook her head no, she did not want to try.

Okay. She would try.

"It's good. I will have a second bite if I can get dessert."

"Your daughter is ridiculously charming." The agent dabbed a napkin into her water glass, wiped sauce from Lily's chin.

"She spends a lot of time with adults," I said.

"Well, it's really paid off."

"Can I have cake?" Lily asked.

"To Lily." Glamber raised her glass for a toast. "More socially at ease at four than I am as a grown woman."

We emerged from the restaurant into light rainfall, the sky a special effect of unholy gray, the streets empty except for random stragglers. I fastened Lily back into the stroller, rolled out its little plastic guard. Her eyes were drooping, those chubby cheeks gone a bit slack. Even so, her face was delicate, a bit glowy, as if powered by an inner light that was on low power. It felt odd, this sensation, as if I were detached from myself, floating . . . wait, not floating, but at once detached and appreciative. How special my daughter was. What a fun, great kid.

WIND SHOOK THE panes in our living room, which would have been concerning, except our ceiling also shook if the upstairs neighbors forgot to take off their shoes. "What's some extra rattle?" I said. Besides, the rainfall didn't seem serious. All those biblical expectations, this monster hurricane was looking like one big blumpo. "We'll be just fine," I said. We went in for bedtime and I left the television on in the living room, believing that Lily was already weary, she'd fall asleep quick, and I could catch the end of the Knicks game. Another example of how little I understood about kids. As was the case after so many major nights, my daughter felt both affectionate and needy. She clung to my arm, asking me to read another story, working to extend the festivities for as long as she could. She rested her head on my chest; strands of her hair scratched my cheek. We cued up twenty-one-year-old Julie Andrews singing live, in black-and-white, "In My Own Little Corner," from a 1957 broadcast of *Cinderella*.

When I came out of the bedroom, the television had gone dormant. In fact, all the lights—including the cable box signal and those little green doodads at the ends of the cord breakers—were off. If a different shade of night hadn't been coming in through the windows, the darkness would have been uniform, impenetrable through the apartment. Flipping switches brought no response. Opening the laptop, however, provided some screen glow. The router was dead and there was no internet, but I wrote for a little bit: Why not take advantage of the lack of possible distractions? Then I thought to keep the charge, put the computer to sleep. Same for my cell.

I'd kept payments on my landline, in part for emergencies like tonight, but with the emergence of smartphones, all the major phone companies had been ignoring the city's physical wiring, meaning my landline had no dial tone. Thank goodness I still had my trusty source for Mets games and late-night sports talk: my seventies-era transistor radio. Fiddling its knob to a news station, I heard about the storm's impact on the East Coast. I heard that a malfunctioning generator on Fourteenth Street blew out the power throughout downtown, even into the east side of Midtown.

I found the two long flashlights I'd bought from one of the police supply stores next to the precinct on the other side of Third, unscrewed their bottoms, loaded each one with new batteries. I also unwrapped a small square light; attached to a head strap, it looked like something a child from a previous century would wear going down into a coal mine. Why would a police supply store have a kid's coal-mining flashlight? Fucking Manhattan is why. Terrified parents who bend over backwards when prepping for emergency situations, is why.

The next morning, Tuesday, the apartment looked pretty much like it always did, except for the dead cable box and cord breaker lights. We dressed like normal. I explained that school was canceled, but we couldn't play computer games right now. I tried to get Lily to eat some cold cereal and bananas, loaded supplies into my backpack. We put on our jackets, grabbed the stroller. I crouched to a knee, waited for her to meet my stare.

"We're going on an adventure," I said. "We're going to see what's going on outside. "

Three fingers in her mouth, she looked up at me.

"So we need to stay together. You need to follow instructions."

She blinked, kept staring.

"You know the rules for the bus station? How we act at the airport?"

It took some time and effort to rise from out of my crouch; I ended up using the folded stroller for help, turning it into a complex walking stick. Lily got distracted by this; I could see her taking in my struggle.

All the overhead hallway lights were silent, their usual hum quieted. The elevator was similarly dead.

Four winding flights awaited, a black yawning mouth.

"Okay, we're watching our steps, right?"

Lily nodded, waited. Now a tentative attempt; she yelped, pulled back. "It's dark. It's *scary*."

Right. My accident in the lobby. Almost two years previous.

I started to say it was all right, she could do it.

Before the words got out, my good little soldier flipped on her headlamp. A Popsicle of light erupted atop her noggin.

"Hey hey." The hall echoed with smacking sounds, my hands pounding together. "Ready Freddie and our aim is steady."

"*Correct-a-mundo, Little Bundo,*" she announced, and turned the light off, back on, showing me how it worked. Her smile was wide and toothy, letting loose another zillion kilowatts.

THE ONLY TIME you saw people walking down the middle of Third Avenue in Manhattan was during a street festival, when police closed off the street with traffic barriers and there were food trucks and food trailers and booths for socks and crafts and phone carriers, and pedestrians wandered between them all, eating greasy junk, occasionally buying some trinkets or a shirt with a graffitied mailbox on it. Lily loved these festivals; bouncy castles and bottles filled with colored sand were her particular favorites. But this wasn't any kind of festival; it was like nothing I'd seen before. Stores on each side of the street were uniformly shuttered; meanwhile, the avenue itself was filled with people. Imagine that a giant shock wave had emptied out every single building in the neighborhood, and in some kind of parade gone wrong, everyone who lived within however many blocks was outside, packed here on the street, sort of like a zombie movie, only cognizant zombies, looking around, wandering together, as if part of a collective daze, everyone unsure of what was happening, whether we were all moving into a new, unknown reality. It was more than a little ominous: dread seemed everywhere, worry was palpable—though, thankfully, full panic hadn't started. Gossip was spreading, news was getting out: the subways were down; the lower half of the city was powerless; Brooklyn was riots galore.

I double-checked, making sure Lily was locked into the stroller. She followed my lead and checked her safety straps, just to be double-safe sure. I kissed her forehead; her eyes met mine, in this moment sharing all sorts of things she did not have the ability to say: that she did not know exactly what was going on; that she recognized whatever was happening as not normal; that she did not know if she should be worried; that she was worried, wanted reassurance, wanted to hear everything would be okay. How much of a toddler's world moves between safety and the unknown to begin with, between an inner cocoon, that zone where you are secure and all needs are met, and everything out there, all that is waiting to be discovered? What we were doing was clearly beyond her understanding.

"Have you ever visited an aquarium?" I asked.

She looked at me. "What's an aquar-um?"

"Where all the fish and sharks and dolphins live."

She kept staring.

"So wouldn't visiting an aquarium be as new as this?"

I'd confused her enough to calm her, some, which was fine by me. Maybe it would keep her from getting scared. We headed north, crossing Twenty-Sixth, and as I pushed the kid over cracks and ruts in the pavement, I tried to make sure she had a smooth ride, to not run the front wheels of the stroller up into the heels of the man trudging ahead of us. Person after person kept holding up their phone. I couldn't understand, then got it: making it onto a new block meant another effort at getting a signal; it meant renewed disappointment with your carrier.

I thought of Cormac McCarthy and *The Road*, specifically the dad guiding his boy through the apocalypse. I couldn't help myself. I similarly remembered Saramago's *Blindness*, the horrible part where every member of society is thrust into blackness. More digressive thoughts kicked in, more dystopian moments: the movie *Children of Men*, where Clive Owen tries to hide the pregnant woman at the refugee compound; and that Elie Wiesel novel from high school, in which the narrator is forced to let his father die, so he might survive the concentration camp.

That dad-as-Nazi poem.

Grim grim grim. Nothing the slightest bit helpful came to mind. Someone accidentally knocked me from behind, apologized. I said "No problem" but felt myself getting agitated.

If the crowd became a mob, what was my game plan?

How would I protect my child if punches were thrown?

If the lights didn't come back on for a while and food turned scarce?

What was our escape?

If I'm distracted by someone, if I look to my phone for an alert—if I go piss against a wall—

Some demented fuck takes the stroller and zips.

Some half-witted perv waves a lollipop.

One second everything fine; the next, no way back.

But then it also occurred to me, there had been this *Saturday Night Live* sketch. One of those weird, limit-pushing sketches that comedy writers moon about, and that always get saved for the end of the show (when nobody is watching). For whatever reason— let's say a counter to my worst-case, Nazi-in-verse scenarios—I thought of it.

Will Ferrell and Joan Cusack were the co-hosts of a morning talk show. The teleprompter went on the fritz. Asked to ad lib, Ferrell and Cusack panicked. "I had a notion the other day," Ferrell said. "I was thinking someone should get together a group with guns to clean out those ghettos." When they cut to the weatherman, David Alan Grier was also panicking, staring at the screen. Before long, Will Ferrell had overturned the set. He and the weatherman wrestled for dominance. Ferrell drank blood from the weatherman's decapitated head. Then the teleprompter started working again. The crisis was over.

As mentioned earlier, I have no talent as a cartoonist; if I did, here is another place I would insert a drawing, done as if from a children's book—let's say a fancy, thin-lined style often used in picture books about young girls. This drawing would show me pushing a stroller down a city street. In the backdrop, gloomy towers, looming brownstones. Zombies in the street. The child is happy, checking out everything. Meanwhile I am thinking:

The teleprompter gets fixed.

If I don't freak out, she won't freak out.

Things will get fixed.

Foot traffic backed up; crowds began to clump. I veered us out of the pedestrian flow. A small crowd had started gravitating toward one side of the street. As we got closer, the storefront's signage became apparent: brick oven pizza. Right—brick ovens didn't need electricity, explaining why the metal gate was rolled back, the shop open.

Yankees cap, Starter jacket, handsome, emerged from the shop, two paper plates held above his head. "They totally jacked the price," he announced, breaking into the recognizable patois of a bond trader who enjoys listening to Wu-Tang. *"But this shit is gooood."*

"Thirsty?" I asked.

Lily nodded. I reached into my backpack, pulled out our water bottles.

I dug deeper, looking for some fruit leather. While scrounging around the bottom of my bag, I grabbed the transistor radio.

News sports and weather on the ten had nothing new to report.

Same with National Public. Corporate newscasts. Sports and weather on the FAN. Nobody so much as estimated when the lights might come back on.

"Someone, please tell us when this will be fixed," I said.

"They must have told the news to not bring up any time frames," said a voice behind me.

"It's in the public interest to not panic us; we're just plebes."

"The juice has to come on, though." I looked back at them, wanting affirmation. "Tribeca, the Village, Gramercy, Flatiron—these are big-ticket neighborhoods. That's the whole point of privilege." I sort of laughed. "Their fancy umbrellas should protect me and my kid on something like this. The cavalry comes for the rich folk, suctions out some water, duct-tapes the circuits—"

I turned to my left, looked around.

Adults. Bodies. Where—

"Lily?"

Turned to my right.

"LILY?"

An announcer was letting the world know that Wall Street and the Nasdaq had both been suspended for the day. The two good people who had been eagerly volunteering their opinion about the government also started looking around, searching with me. An ambulance siren was going off not too far away.

Someone was asking, "Where did you see her?" Someone else was saying, "He can't find his kid."

"I . . ."

"She was right—"

The street had a slight grade to it. I started looking between people.

And saw something.

Maybe a first down away, near the sidewalk. Might have been a triangle. That familiar shade of yellow.

But couldn't see the whole thing.

The fit body of that Starter jacket bro was in the way, putting the finishing bites to his slice.

"LILY."

I sprinted, my footsteps pounding through my ears.

"She yours?"

I didn't answer, veering around him. The sky above was slate and ice. Static from my radio carried.

The stroller's front wheels had indeed banked against the side of the curb. I ran around to the front.

Beneath the fabric's canopy, Lily was strapped in, safe, her face fresh and slick, her eyes oblivious.

"You got to use the brake on these things." From behind me.

I caught my breath, "I swear to Christ I was, not ten seconds ago—"

His hand on my shoulder. "Seriously, though," he said. "Boss, how awful would that have been, losing your kid in the middle of all this?"

His face was concerned and well-meaning, maybe a tinge of judgment.

In my mind, cops were cuffing me, pushing my head into a patrol car; the bro was bent over, his nose broken, streaming blood.

I felt control giving way, curled my hands into fists.

Two years now: two years of the bizarre stray shit gathering in my pockets; two years of that baby violin screeching out noises that made dogs howl, the wasted dead time in a freezing emergency room, the barroom brawls about brushing her teeth, my worst instincts, my worst feelings about myself, the bile, the venom, storing up, biding time, working out, getting stronger, just waiting its turn, waiting to be proven right. Incalculable mental energy, and the sad truth is, unquantifiable amounts of it had been generated through my anticipation of whatever new disaster *had to be* waiting, just around the next corner. Would this disaster be the larger world sweeping in, doing its horrors? Would I be the one who snapped, finally translating my worries about my lack of parental acumen into a self-fulfilling prophecy? What would ignite the next explosion? How would it happen?

I'd been on guard just minutes ago. Hell, this whole book long, you've been reading half worried. Was this going to be the fuse?

Now. *Now.*

From somewhere down below my waist, I felt a pulling, the end of my jacket.

Hair was tangled all over her forehead, and still the fineness of her bone structure was apparent along her temples, her mother's paleness glowing out at the world.

This frail wisp of a thing; looking up at me, her eyes overly girlish but sensing an unease—more, even.

"If there's a problem . . . ," Lily began.

We'd come to another fork in the road. And I could see that Lily was doing her best to veer her old man.

Doing her best to get herself to someplace better.

Gears inside me ratcheted; pulleys tightened.

I welled up, swallowed.

"Yo," I said.

"I want to walk," Lily said. She jerked her seat now, shaking the chassis. "I want to go to the playground."

In my head, Lily was watching me get driven off by cops. What then? If I got charged with assault, would she go to child family services? An orphanage?

I called out thanks. If the bro heard, he did not respond, kept on shrinking into the street scene.

"You've been in there awhile." I wiped sweat from my brow. "You've got to be squirmy. Need to pee?"

Harder shakes to the stroller. "I want to play."

"We're going to find somewhere for you. Just hang in, okay?"

Lily's eyes sharpened. Her focus honed and narrowed. I recognized that she did not have the words for what she wanted to say. Right now she wanted so much more than words, wanted *out*, wanted *action*, she was *eager*.

But also was doing something else.

She chewed her thumb knuckle. Her cheeks sucked inward. She considered.

"I will hang in."

WHEN WE ARRIVED back in our neighborhood, it was just starting to get dark, the overcast sky turning gloomy. A little foot traffic, not much, nobody walking dogs, a patina of normalcy to the street, the familiarity of what is known. Thank hell. We were fried by then. Swings and a really good jungle gym; the discovery of a bank vestibule where the juice was still flowing and people were lined up to recharge their phones and laptops. (I withdrew five twenties, future insolvency taking a back seat to present-day apocalypse.) We'd seen a four-story apartment building with its front sliced away like a birthday cake. (On one high floor was half of a cluttered bedroom, an exposed closet of clothes, the raw power of nature. "A dollhouse," Lily said. "A giant could reach in and play house.") We'd also hit the Times Square Toys"R"Us (dolly stroller, lollipops, liquid bubble mix), then found a food truck on Twenty-Fifth for a hot dinner—chicken tacos and rice, eaten beneath the sky's pastel colors. Now my thighs and calves burned. The bottoms of my feet felt as if I'd ground glass into them.

Lily had caught her sixth wind, though. She was balancing herself on the ledge of a brick flower bed. She was running the block, jumping up and down on different brownstone steps. She blew and chased bubbles. She raced her new dolly stroller back and forth in front of our building. She meandered, reaching for leaves from low branches. I sat on the stoop, watched, appreciated.

A longtime resident was rolling her travel suitcase out of our building. "I found a hotel room uptown," she said, then headed to the curb, tried hailing a cab.

It seemed clear: most of the neighborhood had bailed. Should we?

The humid evening provided no answers.

Cut to upstairs. We're in our bedclothes, cozy under the covers. Lily took her familiar position, nestled into my side, leaning the back of her head on my chest, just below my shoulder.

But was still jittery, couldn't stay in place. I put the compact disc of *Singin' in the Rain* into my laptop, called up one of her favorite songs—Debbie Reynolds busting out of the cake.

"No," she said, rocking left to right.

"How about 'Make 'Em Laugh'?"

"I don't want that."

I ran through songs; she did not want songs. I tried *Sesame Street*; she did not want *Sesame Street*. I asked what she wanted. She didn't know what she wanted.

"*Jeremiah was a bullfrog,*" I began, off-key as usual.

Lily started crying, clawed her nails into my side.

"It makes sense if you are freaked. You did a great job keeping it together."

"*No,*" she said.

"It's been a *very* long day. This blackout is hard. Everyone's having problems."

Fully melting down now, bawling.

"Okay, do you have any ideas?"

"*NO. NO.*"

"*Hey.*" I felt myself starting to lose it. "You're not the only one who had a long day."

"NOOO."

I took a breath, then another. Maybe there was something special I could show her, something to comfort her?

"No," Lily repeated.

"Hold on a sec," I said.

"NO."

I called up a few other files from the hard drive. *Just hold on, goddamn it."*

PEOPLE ASK WHETHER Lily has any memories of her mom. Simple bottom-line answer: No. Freud posited that none of us have memories from before age three, and this statement basically holds true with all adults. It definitely holds with children, specifically with Lily. No conscious memories, no tactile recall, zero.

However, there's also a more complex formulation, one that takes a bit to unpack.

It's worth remembering: when Diana got pregnant—back during the Paleolithic era of 2008—more than a few insightful people were suspicious about the wide-scale cultural effect of smartphones. Attention spans and inner lives were going to be put at risk, went the thinking: resistance was important. This argument has turned out to be both true and immaterial. The future futured forward; we are where we are; even the dumbest of smartphones has capacities well beyond any single mortal's imagination, and the cell phone isn't just accepted, but is a necessity for daily life in our half-civilized twenty-first century.

Back in the aughts, though, Diana and I had committed to the team with books and internal rumination. Which is a pretentious way of saying we consciously decided to be behind the technological curve. Diana had a cell phone, but the kind where every number on the keypad corresponded to three possible letters for texting. I didn't even have that: no cell for me, not until after Lily was born, when we both conceded, okay, it was important to reach one another on short notice. We purchased BlackBerries and, you guessed it, immediately took to our new toys, filling our phones' limited memory cards with pictures of the infant, as well as ten to twenty videos.

Some are all of three seconds. A few are as long as two minutes. Every video is grainy. Every one of them focuses on the baby. We parents are outliers, other people are extras. I report this for context.

When Diana was diagnosed with leukemia, our focus, as I've mentioned, turned to that fight. During which time, we applied a certain approach to the disease. This approach was something I'd learned back in my twenties, when I lucked into two seasons covering a professional football team as a beat writer for a small newspaper. The coach and players constantly fielded *if* questions from us media: If the 49ers beat the Rams, that makes Sunday an elimination game. What would that mean for the franchise? The answers were always the same: We don't deal with hypotheticals. We can only focus on the game we have to play.

At my urging, Diana and I adopted this attitude: Let's worry about what's in front of us.

Even at the end, planning out and filming something for Lily, a speech or address—whether on a mobile phone or a camcorder—would have felt like an acknowledgment, admission that none of the herbal remedies, the meditation and yoga, the chemo and radiation, the experimental drugs, the whole chimichanga—none of it—was going to work.

I want to write that our focus was so great, our confidence so high, that we couldn't even acknowledge that it was natural, *human*, at certain moments, to look beyond the fight. But this would not be true. Our fear was just so large. How could we stare into it? Yet we did, sort of.

There were two conversations about Diana's wishes for after she passed. She also left me letters—one saying what she hoped for me, one with instructions about what she wanted after her passing—and also a letter that Lily is supposed to read later, when she's older: fifteen or sixteen will be the appropriate age.

We also talked about filming a video message Lily could watch later in her life. But we never filmed it. Too great a breach of our faith, I guess.

The truth is, most of our attention and energies and work went into keeping her around.

A long way of saying: there are just a few videos of Diana and her daughter together.

A glance at the laptop's battery icon showed it to be middling, more than capable.

I didn't tell Lily what I was doing, just asked her—once more— to watch.

I double-clicked.

May 23, 2010: After the first transplant, taken by Diana's mother during Diana's first remission. A video of the baby. She is one and a half, playing on the floor of our apartment. Diana's head and body are in the shot for a few seconds via a snippet: the bottom of her chin and most of her neck; they look pale, dry, and doughy, decades older than Diana's real age (thirty-nine at the time). Diana is sitting in her desk chair, watching the child. She is beaming, hugely entertained by her little girl.

Lying in that familiar part of the bed, which she thought of as *hers*, assumed to be *hers*, looking like an impossible, miniature incarnation of her mother, Lily did not move. Her mouth hung open.

She had seen it before, but not many times.
Not enough times.
She sat up.
"Again," she said.
We watched again.

June 25, 2010: Lily, still one and a half. Diana is back in Memphis, having gotten approval for the trip, thanks to reasonably clean test results. Jacuzzis are against doctor's orders but there isn't much chance of her staying out of her aunt and uncle's backyard hot tub. Diana is in the water; also in the water, her aunt, uncle, and Lily. Diana's hair is black, short, and curly, in all ways different than the brown shag she had before the transplant, taking the hair and fingernail characteristics of your donor being one of the effects of a bone marrow transplant. Diana is wearing granny glasses, smiling. A wet T-shirt loosely covers her frame, which is skeletal at best. In her lap she holds Baby Lily beneath those chubby baby arms. Lily is all skin and skull, possessing only a slick cowlick of hair. Diana's uncle and aunt are lightly tossing small plastic balls at Lily, who picks up and bites down on a yellow ball. A red one. "Baaaw. Baaw," Lily squeals. Delighted, she examines the balls. Holding the camera, Peg asks if Lily got water in her eye. Lily answers, "Yeah," then splashes. Diana reaches and helps Lily balance. Lily plays peekaboo with her uncle. Diana watches them—again, enthralled.

Lily scooted upward, into a sitting position. The comforter fell in front of her. She cared not a whit.

"Another one," she said.

November 26, 2011: two weeks before Diana died. Sitting in her desk chair, facing into our living room. Her hair is brown scrub. A yellow paper mask covers the bridge of her nose and her mouth. She's wearing pajamas, a pink robe. In her lap, unsuspecting Toddler Lily, resplendent in a yellow blouse and purple pants with flowers. Mother and daughter look across the room, to our television screen—the part of *The Wizard of Oz* where the world's just gone color. Dorothy is arriving in Oz, receiving those famous sung orders: "*Follow the yellow brick road.*"

The child is enrapt. Diana watches as well. Neither moves. The sounds from the television are faint.

THE THREE CLIPS combined lasted maybe a minute and fifteen seconds. Nothing, really. The last one, the "*Wizard of Oz*" clip, wasn't even thirty seconds. It had been too hard for me to stand there and film, had felt voyeuristic, maybe even predatory. I'd watched it only maybe four times since Diana had passed. It always acted like an atom bomb upon me. I mean, they all hurt, made me feel like heading into bed and curling into a ball for a few hours. But this last clip—we'd been on the cusp of so much: Diana, Lily, me, each of us with our fates just ahead. Diana had to know it, and how could this have been anything but terrifying? Even then, I knew my wife well enough to understand that, seated in that chair, she was channeling all of her strength and soul to stay in that moment, to just sit and appreciate that time, those seconds with her girl.

Tonight, though, I did not feel blown to shreds. Anything but.

"I think that's what we got," I said. "*Oh—*"

Searching through my hard drive, different keywords. "Wait," I said—

Diana as a teenager, back during the eighties, part of the cast for this, a homemade horror film, done with her friends. She is young, lithe, and has a frizzy perm, cotton candy hair that seems, if not exclusive to, then claimed by Southern women of the time. A bit of typecasting: Diana plays the pie-eyed optimist. She has one line of dialogue, which, I remember now, we always enjoyed repeating to one another: "The world is a mixed-up and crazy place, and we just have to accept people for who they are."

"Yes," I said, then remembered something else. "Right." Clickity click.

That one clip from her pregnancy, taken at the baby shower she had with her friends. Diana had long wanted to learn the famed dance from Michael Jackson's *Thriller*. In this clip, she is front and center and blimp pregnant, surrounded by the friends she loves. Everyone moves to the left, points, moves to the right. Diana is a bit behind, a bit slow. She's having the time of her life.

I hadn't ever thought of showing them. I can't quite tell you why: most likely I hadn't believed Lily was old enough to understand them. Next to me, she still might not have been old enough to understand, or even follow, the actions. Did it matter? Whether or not Lily could create order from these happenings, they were her mother. *Mom.* Ethereal to her, cosmic, a concept. She hadn't known it was possible to even consider her mother as a person, let alone to witness Diana as flesh and blood—a teenager trying to act, a pregnant woman laughing as she danced behind the beat.

Lily stared at the screen, waiting for more.

I clicked that file shut. My heart was pumping pretty good, another moment when I wasn't completely in control. The photos were painful but also filled me with momentum, made my hands move quicker, my thumb directing the laptop mouse pad. I made little throaty noises, found the proper folder, started going at it, opening photos—from BlackBerrys, T-Mobile Sidekicks, photos sent from friends' iPhones: Diana and the swaddled newborn;

Diana and the moon-eyed, mostly bald baby; Diana and the not-quite-bald-anymore infant—the growing little girl with the massive forehead that Diana schlepped in her baby carrier while she taught. They opened in a flash and I got a straight snapping jab, not just the memory, but all the attendant information, in this case when Diana was first diagnosed, that summer in New Hampshire. The image was Mommy in her hospital bed, cuddling Lily, both of them happy, gorgeous, bald. What also came with it: the doctor and me talking outside the nurses' station, him explaining the complexity of the disease, Diana, later that morning, asking me to find an organic market where they might have all-natural baby formula.

Hundreds of these. There had to be. Almost three years' worth of photos.

I showed another one to Lily now: this is what your mommy looked like; this is what your mommy did with you. I wanted her to see it all, to know everything.

Here is what Mommy did. And here you are with your mother; this is what you did.

Again and again Lily witnessed what had already been so apparent: Lily did indeed have a mommy. And no matter how tired Mommy might have been, no matter what horrid treatment she'd just been through, the woman in the pictures was overjoyed to be with her daughter: that joyous spirit present, her love for her child bursting through.

This. This is what we had, all the memories that I could show, the stories I could repeat—

And the stories that Grandma Peg would be telling, like about Diana falling off a horse when she was six and breaking her arm.

And the stories from her godmom, Susannah, and from all of Diana's other friends and relatives.

If we looked at enough pictures and watched enough videos and told all the stories—if we created new memories, imprinted new ideas—who knows? Maybe . . .

The little girl was yawning. She shut her eyes, seemed snug beneath the comforter, ready for sleep, giving in. Then she opened them, just barely, the thinnest slits. A satisfied look. Lily reached out, her hand almost making it around my wrist. "When I wake up tomorrow," she said, "I think the lights will be on."

CHAPTER ELEVEN

LILY'S PREDICTION TURNED out to be wrong. The lights and electricity remained dormant, our apartment cold and dull.

I poured out some dregs of dry cereal for her, tried to get a handle on just what kind of playing field we'd be dealing with. From the transistor radio, the news was as follows: the metropolitan subway system had flooded, with the MTA chairman calling the hurricane "the most devastating event in the history of the 108-year-old system." Local schools were still canceled. The Halloween parade too. "Trick or treating will happen another day," I said. I mentioned that she still had all her candy from the West Village festival. "That's something, right?"

Lily's flat expression meant she understood each word but did not want to accept their collective meaning, their inherent truth. She shivered, the glazed bricks of this old building were acting as an incubator for the morning's cold.

Without power, chill and gloom solidified this apartment as a dead zone. Staying put wasn't an option. "All right," I said. "We have more adventure ahead of us today." Oddly enough, I felt a rush as I spoke, found myself believing my words, looking forward to figuring this out. My mind started: the radio had just made clear that subways were out, which meant fewer options for us; anywhere we'd go had to be via foot, maybe a taxi, if I could find one. I began to triangulate: visits to that bank vestibule would allow us to recharge, meaning I no longer had to parcel out my phone and computer usage. Which meant: *okay, open the laptop.*

This is how I discovered that the late-night mass email I'd sent—from my phone, asking anyone for playdates—had received untold responses. A list of parents from Third Street. One or two dashed-off sentences at a time, mostly good wishes. Like the majority of our building's residents, they'd already fled the city. My sitter had checked in to cancel her scheduled visit, which made sense: Who'd expect her to show up in the middle of this? Friends also were touching base. Buses were beginning to run over the Brooklyn Bridge: Did we want to take one and use an extra room in Park Slope?

Down my inbox I clicked, considering each offer, my universe expanding with goodwill, even that cheesiest of words, "gratitude."

Then I saw A's name. Our first contact since I'd ended things.

It hurt her to think of us being without power. She did not know if I even had access to email, and she did not want me getting wrong ideas. Her roommate was stuck upstate. I was encouraged to take Lily and get into a taxi. We could shower, recharge the batteries, nap. If necessary, Lily and I could take her bed. She would sleep on the couch.

It's gorgeous, a kind and selfless gesture, arriving directly out of some classic, much-anthologized short story. All I had to do was take the invitation, grab us a taxi, take A up on her kindness. Just ride up into Queens and tear off that scab. If I didn't want to do that, then a variant of the concept: move in the opposite direction, ordering the cab across the Brooklyn Bridge, into Fort Greene. We could ride things out with the nice married couple who hung out with Lily on Saturday nights.

Manhood. Just what does it mean to be a man? There have been lofty notions: responsibility and duty have been thrown around a decent amount, especially with regard to fatherhood. But let's be honest: Men also might have an ego and insecurity at the same time, which results in a territorial lack of familiarity with other boroughs. Men might not want to impose. Men might not want to be at the mercy of people they don't know all that well. Men might refuse to be put in *more* emotional debt, or might just respond to the gut instinct that says, *Nah.* Men need to prove shit to themselves. Men have martyr complexes. Men separate themselves, alienate themselves, refuse to read writing that all but glows from on the wall. Men ignore people who, out of the blue, because they are concerned for a little girl, emailed. Men, or some men—or one man—decide, *We can play this to the end.*

I did not answer A's email. Lily turned down both of the outfits I'd selected for her. Instead, she walked directly to her chest of drawers, selected her own clothing. I let her pack a baggie of her favorite Halloween candy, pretended I did not see her sneak that miniature-sized Milky Way, the lump of chocolate in her cheek. Final dregs of Pirate's Booty, *check.* Quarters from Change Lake, *check.* Helping ease her feet down through her tights, helping her get into her jacket sleeves, securing her backpack, *checkity check check.*

"Do we have to?" she asked.

"You just take your time, turn on your light." I locked both locks on the front door. "Just like yesterday," I said. "You'll do great."

Halfway between the second and first floor, she became rigid. Extending her arms, Lily shook her hands out in front of her. Her breaths were deep; color flooded to her face.

"What?" I asked.

She summoned her courage: "I don't want you to fall again."

"Don't worry," I said. "Daddy's good."

"No." Her voiced echoed through the stairwell. "When you were running and fell and had to go to the hospital. It was my fault."

I heard my pulse in my ears. I put my hands on the sides of her head, took my time brushing down her hair. I smiled at her, kissed her forehead.

"Listen to me," I said. "You were three. You couldn't have done anything bad."

Her eyes stayed with mine. Her breathing seemed to calm.

"We were playing," I said. "It just happened. It was an accident. Whoopsie."

She nodded just a bit. She seemed to hear. Her cheeks were red, shining wet.

I sensed it wasn't over; there was still something wrong. I maintained our eye contact, kept looking at her, kept breathing.

"Mommy?" I asked.

Lily gave another little nod.

"I can't stop thinking of the videos." Her words came out all at once, almost a shout. "It *is* my fault."

"No."

"*It is.*"

"Mommy just got sick," I said. "Everyone tried to help her. The doctors tried. Everyone who loves Mommy tried."

I touched my forehead to hers. "It could not be your fault." I tapped my head against hers a second time. "She lived for *you*. You are her baby."

Again I said, "She lived for *you*."

With this, Lily's shoulders heaved. Something inside her gave way, loosening, not becoming undone—not that—but something inside her unclenched, softening. She was still sobbing, her face was a mess, a crimson rictus, at once pain and relief. But that was okay. "I live for you," I said. "Daddy lives for you too."

Lily responded by touching the top of her head to my forehead. We pressed into each other and then she slipped off and leaned into my shoulder, burrowing, digging her face into the rough fabric of my sample sale coat. She released a snort, staying in my shoulder for a time, until, with what almost seemed a shyness, she withdrew, a bit, and wiped her snot on my collar.

THE BLACKOUT WOULD last another four days, ending early Friday evening, when, with little warning, the lights and television went back on inside the apartment.

We couldn't know this on that morning, of course.

What we could know—what we could *do*—was this:

On the front step of our apartment building that last morning of October, with the clouds breaking and patches of faint blue peeking through along the rim of sky, I could reach out my hand to Lily. Lily could put her thin little fingers around the tattoo on my ring finger. We could stand there; electricity could run through her thin little fingers; nuclear power could run through my tattooed ring finger. Our connection could throb through our veins, could pulse through our hearts, could erupt through our bodies. Ahead of us, we had the day, the city, the world, leaves, the wind; we had the universe, the known, the mystical, the metaphysical, the profane, the profound— all ahead of us, waiting.

In a Zen tale, a young monk, brand-new to a monastery, asks how he can help, what he can do. An older monk asks, "Have you eaten?" The younger monk nods. Says the older monk: "Wash your pot."

Do the next right thing is that idea.

I could call my sister and see how she and her kids were doing. I could strap Lily into the stroller and wheel her across Lexington Avenue and come upon a crew from Con Ed at work around a man-hole and ask if they'd figured out what was wrong and have them say, *Not a clue.* I could push the stroller across the west side of Union Square, where the farmers market usually was, and come upon a fleet of parked utility company trucks and ask how long it was going to take to get the lights back and get the same shrug that those workers were giving the other thousand people who'd asked in the last hour.

Superdad here hadn't taken care of laundry before the storm. Lily and I were both tattered, needing showers. Potentially, we could finish with my sister and head north, toward the flagship Macy's on Thirty-Fourth. Once there, I could procure Lily packs of underwear and socks. She could try on a few cute outfits. I could find snow boots in her size blessedly on sale.

Ahead lay her first haircut. Ahead lay her first loose tooth. One particularly terrible Mother's Day I'd take her to a dance recital to get her away from all the festivities, and the ushers would make a point of handing a red rose to every mom in attendance.

Today, though, what else could we do? Well, on our way back from Macy's, potentially we could take in a most curious site— indeed, that most New Yorkish of images: the famed modernist skyscraper where King Kong had made his fatal ascent. We could gaze upon the Empire State Building, glowing amid the darkened and closed city block, the iconic tower literally emanating with light, spilling excesses from its store marquees, from untold windows. I could ask someone, and learn that the Empire State Building operated on its own power grid, independent from the rest of the city.

We were ourselves operating on our own power grid, independent of the rest of the city, two little flashlight beams amid this wounded, flickering, kaleidoscopic extravaganza.

How were we going to survive?

How were we going to keep doing this?

Day two of a blackout probably wasn't the time for me to go Vanilla Ice and—*yo*—solve our massive life issues. It was simply time to wash our proverbial pot, to shepherd my daughter through this world in a way that best shielded her from the blackouts, from the disappointments, from maternal absence, from my own inclination toward grouchiness, from my tired spirals, from my desire to have someone listen to and pay attention to me, from my truly dubious decision-making processes, from my endless onslaught of flaws.

We stood in front of our apartment on East Twenty-Second. Our next steps awaited.

We couldn't possibly know what lay ahead. But I looked forward to experiencing it—*all of the great handful that is life*—with my little girl.

EPILOGUE

AS I WRITE this, Lily is thirteen years old, and looks so much like her mom, it often stops me. Her body has filled out into that of a woman; she has braces whose colors get changed with each adjustment, as well as an on-again/off-again Instagram account and hair that she recently dyed a flaming chemical red. She is hell on radioactive wheels. I mean that in the best way: difficult one moment and charming the next, sulking, unreachable, diffident, and then composed, ready to get defensive, go to pieces, or solve a problem at a moment's notice. Like many young women of her day and age, she's hit that place where she wants to spend free time with friends rather than doing things with her dad. She's declared herself to be attracted to girls (my reaction: "*Cool*"), and has declared herself to be beyond gender, putting her foot down about purchasing a man's suit for the first bat mitzvah she'd been invited to. Sometimes I think Lily uses social anxiety as an excuse to act spoiled and pissy, like when the sound of silverware scraping on a plate makes her cry. She recently came home from therapy with Dr. Jennifer Melfi—yes, bless her, Dr. Melfi—and stood in front of me, declaring—with *Fuck you* pulsing through every word—that she was going to get her septum pierced and, whether I liked it or not, I could not stop her, so I might as well support her and let her do it.

I am fifty-three. Lily and I now reside, together, in a different apartment, just a few blocks from where so many of the events of these pages played out. Lily has her own bed now, her own room. We're on the fifth floor of a walk-up, and each time I head up or down all the stairs, I feel it through my knees, especially when I am hauling laundry or groceries. I am still an adjunct professor, nothing more, and fret about what little hair I have left (a *shanda*, how little hair I have left). No home equity. Few stocks. Little savings. Still single. By most of the traditional standards of manhood, I guess I haven't fared so well. At the same time, this last decade has brought a larger societal reconsideration of manhood and what a man is supposed to be, stressed and accentuated the idea of the toxic male, reshaped the traditional white hetero male as a catchall villain, and made clear that the new century's literature and history will not be written by such men. Maybe there's consolation in not meeting such standards, but refashioning them, however microscopically.

FIVE WEEKS AFTER the blackout. We'd started counting down to Lily's fifth birthday. This included a special present for her. I'd been prepping her with a slew of YouTube clips: those black-and-white ones of Julie Andrews, twenty-one years young, live on network television (no way for Julie to know that just around the corner were Mary Poppins and Maria Von Trapp); Leslie Ann Warren in the faded, flowing gowns from her 1965 CBS special. We'd watched the teen star Brandy and the tragic icon Whitney Houston perform their duet (a mid-nineties production, excellent ratings, glowing reviews). Always, we'd returned to one clip, from our current year's Tony Awards broadcast, a medley, Cinderella and her fairy godmother singing about what was and was not possible. The clip transitions into a ballroom dance scene where the prince and Cinderella fall in love with one another from across the room.

Rodgers and Hammerstein's *Cinderella* was on Broadway. In my own slapdash manner, I'd met a guy whose wife had spent her adult life in the theatrical world; she put us in touch with one of the actresses in the Broadway production, one of Cinderella's stepsisters. Lily's birthday fell on a Wednesday, meaning that day had a matinee performance. To celebrate, Lily wore to school a floor-length ball gown costume of white satiny material. She also wore a twinkly plastic tiara. I brought grocery store cupcakes for her classroom celebration, wrote a note informing the school that Lily would be departing early. When I picked her up, she wore a plastic ring; she showed me her new, unsharpened pencil, as well as the other doodads given to her as part of the class birthday packet. Lily was very happy with her gifts—a little too happy for my preference. I double-checked, made sure I had the printout with our tickets.

Our trusty stroller awaited, beaten down at this point, its yellow vinyl no longer bright like sunshine. Still, the wheels—one of which recently had been replaced—rolled just fine. I zipped on her blue winter coat, navigated us out to the avenue, right during the time of day when cabdrivers were changing shifts. It took a while, but we managed to get a taxi. Heading uptown had to be slow, midday traffic horrible—all the clichés of a world that cannot let you have anything nice.

Somewhere around Fortieth and Lex, it was apparent that if we stayed in that cab, we'd be late. I had the driver let us out, unfolded the stroller from the back, and indeed started us off—"Don't worry"— sprinting and pushing Lily in that stroller, swerving along busy Midtown side streets, all the way across town to the West Side. We had about twenty minutes. "We got this," I said.

Arriving at the Broadway Theatre (the theater's actual name!), I was swimming in my own sweat, breathing hard enough to have a heart attack. We had enough time to check the stroller, buzz the concession stand, and—though I did not pony up for merch this time—buy some M&M's and water. Our seats were up near the back of the top of the theater. No time to gawk at gilded what-nots. We took our programs, got our coats off, settled into our seats. I reminded Lily that once the show started, the lights would go down.

"I know," she said.

The moment the show started, she grabbed my hand.

She explained what would happen in the scenes where Cinderella was bossed around by her stepmother.

She was not at all prepared for Prince Charming to slay that giant monster puppet: recoiling, closing her eyes, opening them. She kept watching.

And marveled at the scene in the town square, the complicated dance number involving most of the cast, immaculately choreo-graphed, with invitations to the ball handed out.

When Cinderella sang the famous song—"*In my own little corner / In my own little chair*"—Lily sang along. When the crazy old woman twirled and her dress of rags became a ball gown, Lily's YouTube viewings had her prepared. "*That's the fairy godmother*," her whisper shouted toward me.

Then Cinderella twirled and transformed into her iconic and gorgeous dress of blue and white. Lily was amazed, slamming her hands together repeatedly.

After the show, we waited for the crowd to empty, then followed the email with the instructions. As if we were floating, or perhaps transported by a magic pumpkin, we made it down to the stage door. I gave our names to an usher. He checked my ID, crossed us off a list, and stamped Lily's hand with an official royal handstamp. He took us backstage and told us to wait. An open door nearby showed a room with lots of costumes and thread. The hallway was warm, more than a bit dark.

I don't know how long we stood there. Long enough to talk about our favorite parts, to settle into silence, to stay nervous.

Then a woman came out. Though she was not in costume, we recognized her: one of the stepsisters. She was in jeans and stylish boots and a puffy brown winter coat. She asked if this was Lily. She introduced herself: Anne.

Anne asked: "Did you enjoy the show?"

For a moment my daughter turned shy. Then she said this: "Yes, I did. We watched part of it at bedtime on the computer. I got scared by the monster in the forest but the show wasn't scary. It was wonderful. Your sisters song is one of my favorite."

Anne absorbed the monologue with a smile that I have to believe was genuine.

Leading us behind the massive curtain, she apologized but told us we were not allowed to walk onto the stage. We veered backstage, and learned that the giant monster was made up of hundreds of pieces; sixteen puppeteers were required to work the thing. We learned that the theater was so small that a lot of the cast did not have dressing rooms; they just got dressed backstage, performing quick changes behind a series of black curtains.

Anne led us toward the far side of the stage and a large chalk-board. It was set up as a scoreboard, with a series of columns. The columns tracked how many times someone offstage caught the shoe, how many times someone else put up their hand and blocked the catch. Anne even handed Lily a shoe, asked if she wanted to take a throw, pointing to the makeshift bull's-eye by the wall.

Lily gave a little toss, did not seem disappointed about the landing.

This is when Anne did one last kindness. She headed over to the wall pouches. From a folder she removed a yellow sheet; made of slick plastic, it had been printed up to look like an ancient parchment. All afternoon Lily had been more than composed; she'd been charming—not so much her best self as providing a glimpse of who she might become. Presently, her eyes flashed disbelief. As if blindsided, she exhaled a small breath. "Really?" Lily asked. She reached out. I watched, dumbfounded. It is likely true that musicals are indeed love, but we all know, love is human, love is flawed. Nonetheless, flawed human love, in its purest essence, filled me now. What I was seeing play out was like some odd confirmation of my best intentions, an encapsulation of my fondest dreams: my baby, my girl, her thin fingers accepting an invitation to the ball.

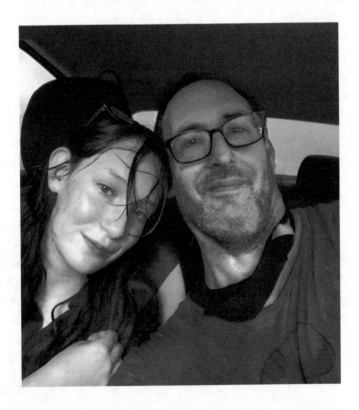

ACKNOWLEDGMENTS

THE TRUTH: A metric ton of people helped me stay alive those early years with Lily. Trying to do justice to them—to thank each person—is as impossible a task as finding a place to write about every one of a child's toys. (No matter how much you try to create space for Rainbow Cube Bot, he still ends up left out.) Still, there was so much kindness toward me. To each of the people who helped, whether you—or specific parts of you—have been shoehorned into these pages or not, please know I remember. I owe you more than I can ever repay.

Another tier: the wondrous people essential to this manuscript getting finished and into the world. This includes but is not limited to Jamie Sears, Said Sayrafiezadeh, John Wray, Ellen Steloff, Mohammed Naseehu Ali, Jaime Clarke, Howard Axelrod, Wyatt Mason, William Lycheck, Adelle Waldman, Gary Shtyngart, Rebecca Makkai, Joanna Rakoff, Tara Ison, Tom Barbash, Bonnie Nadell.

More thanking: Beowulf Sheehan. Ron Yerxa. Albert Berger. A. M. Homes. Sheri Fink. Acacia Shields. John Emerson. Kerry Garfinkel. Isabel Howe and the other largehearted folks at Author's League Fund. Rachel Sopher fixed my brain and laughed at my jokes along the way. Celeste Loft gave us a place to live and has been nothing but kind. Christa Parravani, Bugatti of wisdom and generosity. Joshua Ferris and Matt Thomas, friends to the blood, read many drafts over the years, offered insightful thoughts, and stayed supportive well after they'd justifiably grown sick of these pages, to say nothing of their author. When I was ready to burn this project to ashes, Sean Wilsey saw how the book could not just be salvaged, but maybe become readable. Cressida Leyshon—editorial legend; more than that, a truly kind human—saved more than the day by carving out an excerpt.

Deb Landau, Joanna Yas, Jessica Flynn, and Jerome Murphy at NYU, thank you for giving me a chance to teach. All my students, thank you for putting up with me.

Everyone at Abrams has been a joy to work with. Taryn Roeder is indeed a rock star. Managing editor Lisa Silverman and copyeditor David Chesanow worked out kinks galore and made the prose shine. Thank you to designer Eli Mock and illustrator João Fazenda for the work of art that is the cover (each time I look, it both takes my breath and gets me choked up).

Tina Pohlman's enthusiasm gave me life. Jamison Stoltz, so smart and assured, is a total boss.

I drew fucking aces with Barbara Jones for my literary representation.

Peggy Taylor, you are a blessing; you have given unconditional love and grace. Thank you. Susannah Maurer, the best godmother a child could dream of, you do your best friend's memory proud.

Yale and Anthony Bock are always in my corner, no matter what kind of ass I am. TJ Kenneally is a kind and good man, and breaks the mold as an in-law. Izzy and Declain, lifelong joys. Crystal Kenneally is my bedrock. Caryl Bock taught me that even in the most trying of circumstances, decency is not just possible, but required.

Ione Jamison Bock brings floods of love every single time I see her.

And, of course, my Tomato Tornado. I am so lucky to have spent these years with you, so proud of the person you are becoming.